W9-AVN-777

Dental Office Management

Ellen Dietz, CDA, AAS, BS

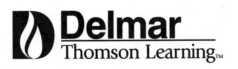

Albany • Bonn • Boston • Cincinnati • Detroit • London • Madrid
Melbourne • Mexico City • New York • Pacific Grove • Paris • San Francisco
Singapore • Tokyo • Toronto • Washington

NOTICE TO THE READER

Publisher does not warrant or guarantee any of the products described herein or perform any independent analysis in connection with any of the product information contained herein. Publisher does not assume, and expressly disclaims, any obligation to obtain and include information other than that provided to it by the manufacturer.

The reader is expressly warned to consider and adopt all safety precautions that might be indicated by the activities herein and to avoid all potential hazards. By following the instructions contained herein, the reader willingly assumes all risks in connection with such instructions.

The Publisher makes no representation or warranties of any kind, including but not limited to, the warranties of fitness for particular purpose or merchantability, nor are any such representations implied with respect to the material set forth herein, and the publisher takes no responsibility with respect to such material. The publisher shall not be liable for any special, consequential, or exemplary damages resulting, in whole or part, from the readers' use of, or reliance upon, this material.

Delmar Staff:

Business Unit Director: William Brottmiller
Acquisitions Editor: Marlene McHugh Pratt
Development Editor: Melissa Riveglia
Editorial Assistant: Maria Perretta
Executive Marketing Manager: Dawn Gerrain

Channel Manager: Nicole Benson
Executive Production Manager: Karen Leet
Project Editor: Bill Trudell
Art/Design Coordinator: Rich Killar
Cover Design: Brucie Rosch

COPYRIGHT © 2000
Delmar is a division of Thomson Learning. The Thomson Learning logo is a registered trademark used herein under license.

Printed in Canada
1 2 3 4 5 6 7 8 9 10 XXX 05 04 03 02 01 00

For more information, contact Delmar, 3 Columbia Circle, PO Box 15015, Albany, NY 12212-0515; or find us on the World Wide Web at http://www.delmar.com

Asia
Thomson Learning
60 Albert Street, #15-01
Albert Complex
Singapore 189969
Tel: 65 336 6411
Fax: 65 336 7411

Japan:
Thomson Learning
Palaceside Building 5F
1-1-1 Hitotsubashi, Chiyoda-ku
Tokyo 100 0003 Japan
Tel: 813 5218 6544
Fax: 813 5218 6551

Australia/New Zealand:
Nelson/Thomson Learning
102 Dodds Street
South Melbourne, Victoria 3205
Australia
Tel: 61 39 685 4111
Fax: 61 39 685 4199

UK/Europe/Middle East:
Thomson Learning
Berkshire House
168-173 High Holborn
London
WC1V 7AA United Kingdom
Tel: 44 171 497 1422
Fax: 44 171 497 1426

Thomas Nelson & Sons LTD
Nelson House
Mayfield Road
Walton-on-Thames
KT 12 5PL United Kingdom
Tel: 44 1932 2522111
Fax: 44 1932 246574

Latin America:
Thomson Learning
Seneca, 53
Colonia Polanco
11560 Mexico D.F. Mexico
Tel: 525-281-2906
Fax: 525-281-2656

South Africa:
Thomson Learning
Zonnebloem Building
Constantia Square
526 Sixteenth Road
P.O. Box 2459
Halfway House, 1685
South Africa
Tel: 27 11 805 4819
Fax: 27 11 805 3648

Canada:
Nelson/Thomson Learning
1120 Birchmount Road
Scarborough, Ontario
Canada M1K 5G4
Tel: 416-752-9100
Fax: 416-752-8102

Spain:
Thomson Learning
Calle Magallanes, 25
28015-MADRID
ESPANA
Tel: 34 91 446 33 50
Fax: 34 91 445 62 18

International Headquarters:
Thomson Learning
International Division
290 Harbor Drive, 2nd Floor
Stamford, CT 06902-7477
Tel: 203-969-8700
Fax: 203-969-8751

All rights reserved Thomson Learning © 2000. The text of this publication, or any part thereof, may not be reproduced or transmitted in any form or by any means, electronics or mechanical, including photocopying, recording, storage in an information retrieval system, or otherwise, without prior permission of the publisher.

You can request permission to use material from this text through the following phone and fax numbers. Phone: 1-800-730-2214; Fax 1-800-730-2215; or visit our Web site at http://www.thomsonrights.com

Library of Congress Cataloging-in-Publication Data
Dietz, Ellen Roberts.
    Dental office management / Ellen Dietz.
        p. cm.
    Includes bibliographical references and index.
    ISBN 0-7668-0731-5
    1. Dental assistants. 2. Office management. I. Title.
RK60.5D54 1999
651'.96176—dc21   99-28104
                                                   CIP

Dedication

Appreciation is extended to Virginia S. Helms, CDA, teacher and friend, to whom this book is dedicated, for her commitment to her students and devotion to dental assisting as a profession. Virginia is Director of Education at the Dental Auxiliary Training Academy, Albuquerque, New Mexico. She has served as past president and past secretary of both the New Mexico Dental Assistants Association and the Albuquerque District Dental Assistants Society.

Ms. Helms is a member in good standing of the American Dental Assistants Association and a past member of the DANB Expanded Functions Test Construction Consultant Committee and is a past member of the Advisory Board to the Dental Department at the University of New Mexico. Ms. Helms is also certified in radiography and is a credentialed Red Cross instructor in CPR and First Aid.

Sharing in This Commitment to Excellence in Education

All royalties from the sale of *Dental Office Management* are designated to a scholarship fund for dental assisting students enrolled full-time in programs that use this text. Scholarships will be awarded annually, based upon need, dedication, and commitment to the dental assisting profession as a career. All inquiries and requests for applications should be directed to the author.

Table of Contents

Preface

Introduction

Dental Office Management was written based upon the need expressed by dental assisting instructors for a comprehensive, detailed and up-to-date text for the front office manager. It is designed for the dental assistant student enrolled in a vocational, proprietary, or post-secondary accredited dental assisting program and is based upon the criteria outlined by the Dental Assisting National Board's *Task Analysis. Dental Office Management* may also be used by on-the-job trained dental assistants and office managers wishing to update their front desk skills or for those dental team members wishing to review for the office management certification examination through the recognized testing pathways.

This text also responds to the needs of the market based upon emerging trends in government regulations, a significant increase in the number of dental practices using computers, the need for proper treatment coding, tighter financial tracking of practice production and expenditures, an increased emphasis on the need for marketing, the emergence of dental managed care programs, and the increasing recognition and responsibilities delegated to the dental office manager.

Organization of the Text

The text is broken down into five sections: *The Business of Dentistry, Practice Communications, Clinical Records Management, Business and Financial Records Management,* and *Employment Opportunities.* Each chapter contains instructional objectives and key terms, which appear in bold throughout. *Italics* has been added to some words for emphasis.

You will also note that there exists frequent cross-referencing of topics throughout this text. This is to enable the student to adequately prepare when comprehension of information from a previous chapter is required before proceeding; also for additional or expanded information on a specific topic.

At the end of each chapter are a *Skill-Building for Success: Student Activity* section and *Skills Mastery Assessment Post-Test*. The skill-building exercises are designed for the student to use critical thinking, problem-solving, and role playing using the information presented in the chapter. These exercises help the student work through practical problem-solving situations commonly encountered in the life of a dental office manager. The post-test is designed in short-answer format for easy recall and quick assessment of information learned in the chapter.

An attempt has been made to reduce gender bias in the preparation of this text. Feedback from the reviewers and publisher resulted in the consensus that while more than 96 percent of dental assistants and office managers are female, references through the text were developed as she/he or the dental office manager.

Acknowledgments

Without the support and encouragement of many wonderful people, this book would not have been possible. I am most grateful for the professional advice and support from the staff at Delmar Publishers and would like to thank Marlene Pratt, Melissa Riveglia, and Maria Paretta, as well as members of the production staff, Bill Trudell, and Rich Killar for their invaluable assistance and encouragement.

Appreciation is also expressed to Gerry Pozzi, my dental assisting teacher, who inspired and encouraged me to pursue dental assisting as a career and beyond; to Dorothy Oldham-Bonner, sponsor of my student teaching and subsequent teaching supervisor and professional mentor; to Kathy Green, professional office consultant, friend, and advisor for her insight, patience, and encouragement in the development of this book; and to John "J.R" Robinson, the gentleman of the dental supply industry.

Appreciation is also extended to the staff of the American Dental Assistants Association, the Dental Assisting National Board, the National Association of Dental Assistants, and the Organization for Safety and Asepsis Procedures (OSAP).

Special thanks are also extended to the numerous dental manufacturers, suppliers, and publishers for generously sharing their product knowledge, photography services, and artwork to enhance the learning experience of students who use this book. Also to the reviewers of this text for their time, dedication, and commitment to excellence in education.

Finally, a word of thanks to my students, past and future, who have taught and inspired me along the way through their shared values, wisdom, and refreshing insights.

The author and Delmar Publishers wish to express their appreciation to a dedicated group of professionals who reviewed and provided commentary at various stages. Their insights, suggestions, and attention to detail were very important in guiding the development of this textbook.

Lori Burch, RDA
Corinthian College
Reseda, California

Robin Caplan, CDA, EFDA, DRT
Medix School
Owings Mills, Maryland

Lana Barnett Edwards, DMD
Lewis and Clark College
Godfrey, Illinois

Darlene Hunziker, CDA, RDA
Eton Technical Institute
Everett, Washington

Barbara Melanson, RDH, MS
Quinsigamond Community
    College
Worcester, Massachusetts

Fred Rich
Gwinett School of Dental Assisting
Lilburn, Georgia

Debbie Reynon, CDA, RDA
Monterey Peninsula College
Monterey, California

Deanne Shuman, BSDH, MS
Old Dominion University
Norfolk, Virginia

About the Author

Ellen Dietz has enjoyed a successful dental career, beginning as an associate-degreed CDA (a graduate of Dutchess County Community College, Poughkeepsie, NY) in private practice. After working as a chairside assistant and office manager, she returned to college and earned her BS in Allied Health Education in Dental Auxiliary Utilization and a Community College Teaching Certificate from the State University of New York at Buffalo.

Following a combined seven-year dental assisting teaching career at Orange County Community College, the University of North Carolina at

Chapel Hill, Erie County BOCES, and Niagara County Community College, she began to pursue her true love, writing about dentistry.

Ellen initially accepted the Front Desk Column of *Dental Assisting Magazine* and one year later took over the managing editor post. In the following years, she worked in dental marketing, project management, and product development at Semantodontics (SmartPractice/SmartHealth) and in legal administration for the Arizona State Board of Dental Examiners. She has published five books in the dental assisting market, was keynote speaker at ADAA Annual Session, and is a licensed business owner.

Ellen has authored numerous accredited continuing dental education home study programs. Her articles have appeared in *JADAA: The Dental Assistant, DENTIST, The Dental Student, Dental Economics, RDH,* and *Dental Teamwork Magazine.* Ellen has also served as editor of *Practice Smart* newsletter *and The Explorer* newsletter. She is a native of upstate New York and resides in Mesa, Arizona.

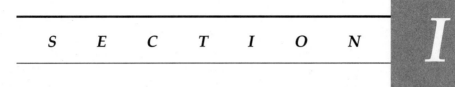

S E C T I O N *I*

The Business of Dentistry

Chapter 1

The Dental Team

- **The Practice Philosophy**
- **The Practice Mission Statement**
- **Serving Patients Is the First Priority**
- **Key Members of the Dental Team**
    The Dentist
    Recognized Dental Specialties
    The Dental Hygienist
    The Dental Office Manager
    The Chairside Dental Assistant
    The Dental Laboratory Technician
    The Denturist
    The Infection Control Coordinator
    Additional Personnel
- **Qualifications and Credentials of the Dental Assistant**
    Licensure and Registration
    Certification
    Eligibility Pathways for Certification
- **Continuing Education**
    Recertification Guidelines
    Continuing Education Audit
- **Working Together as a Team**
    Staff Meetings
    The Morning Huddle
    Goal-Setting
- **Quality Assurance**

Learning Objectives

Upon completion of this chapter, the student will achieve an 80 percent or higher score on the Skills Mastery Assessment Post-Test *covering the following material.*

1. Describe the importance of the practice's philosophy, mission statement, and goals in terms of the dental office manager.
2. List and describe the eight recognized dental specialties.
3. List the educational requirements and job descriptions of the dentist, dental hygienist, dental office manager, chairside dental assistant, and dental laboratory technician; be familiar with extended functions for dental assistants and dental hygienists.
4. List the formal credentials available to the dental office manager and chairside dental assistant, and the requirements for each.
5. List the pathways for certification eligibility.
6. Discuss the importance of continuing education for the dental office manager and chairside dental assistant.
7. Describe the importance of staff meetings and the morning huddle as they relate to all dental team members.
8. Define the perception of quality care as it relates to the dentist and the patient, and the responsibilities of the staff associated with providing it.

Key Terms

anomaly/anomalies

Certified Dental Assistant (CDA)

chairside dental assistant

Dental Assisting National Board
   (DANB)

dental hygienist

dental laboratory technician

dental office manager

dental service representative

dental supply representative

dental office manager

denturist

endodontics

endodontist

esthetics

infection control coordinator

operatory

oral pathologist

Key Terms (cont.)

oral pathology

oral prophylaxis

oral surgeon

oral surgery

orthodontics

orthodontist

pediatric dentist (formerly pedodontist)

pediatric dentistry (formerly pedodontics)

periodontics

periodontist

practice goals

practice mission statement

practice philosophy

prostheses

prosthodontics

prosthodontist

public health dentist

public health dentistry

To ensure a well-run office, the dental office manager must be familiar with the **practice philosophy, practice mission statement,** and resulting **practice goals,** as well as with all duties performed in the office by team members.

The Practice Philosophy

The practice philosophy is the underlying theme that drives the practice on a daily basis. It includes attitudes, delivery of service, patient satisfaction, and quality of service.

The Practice Mission Statement

The practice mission statement is a succinct declaration of the practice philosophy, usually formulated into one or two sentences. An example would be, "To provide the highest quality of dental care and service, and to treat each patient as a welcome guest."

Many offices include the practice mission statement on their statements, letterhead, newsletter masthead, or other printed communications.

Serving Patients Is the First Priority

In any practice, the first priority of the dental team is to serve all patients with courtesy, and a quality, service-oriented philosophy. To accomplish this goal, all members of the team must work cohesively through a communication system of mutual respect. This begins with full knowledge of each team member's role, job description, and educational background.

Key Members of the Dental Team

The following people comprise the dental team.

The Dentist

The dentist must have graduated from a dental school approved by the *Commission on Dental Accreditation of the American Dental Association* and be *licensed* in the state in which he or she practices. (*Note:* Practicing dentistry without a license is subject to disciplinary action before the State Dental Board.) The four-year dental school course of study is preceded by two to four years of undergraduate study in the biomedical sciences.

In addition to holding a license to practice dentistry, the dentist must also have a narcotics license to write prescription medications for patients.

Once a graduate of a dental school, the dentist is addressed as *doctor*. The dentist earns either a *DDS* or *DMD* degree conferred by the school of dentistry.

DDS stands for doctor of dental surgery (although this does *not* mean that the graduate is an oral surgeon); *DMD* stands for doctor of medical dentistry (which does *not* mean that the graduate is a physician). Two-thirds of all dental school graduates become general practitioners. The remaining one-third become dental specialists.

Recognized Dental Specialties

Upon graduation from an accredited dental school, the dentist may elect to pursue additional education credentials in one of the eight recognized dental specialties. Each specialty determines its own educational requirements. Specific testing to earn *Board Certification* may be required.

Once a dentist becomes a specialist, he or she must limit the practice and scope of dental treatment exclusively to that specialty. The eight recognized dental specialties are:

- **Prosthodontics** – the field of restoration and maintenance of normal dentition and its functions through replacement with artificial teeth. A **prosthodontist** is a dental specialist who replaces lost natural teeth with fixed **prostheses** (crowns, bridges, or implants) or removable prostheses (full or partial dentures).

- **Periodontics** – the field of preserving natural tooth structures through disease prevention and treatment of the supporting tissues of the teeth. A **periodontist** is a dental specialist who performs gingival (gum) treatments, including surgery, exposure of oral implants, and occlusal (chewing) adjustments.

- **Oral surgery** (including maxillofacial surgery and reconstruction) – the field of diagnosis and treatment of diseases and malformations of the oral cavity and surrounding structures. An **oral surgeon** is a specialist who extracts teeth, removes diseased tissue, surgically exposes impacted teeth, wires fractured jaws, and places dental implants. A *maxillofacial surgeon* may also treat victims of automobile accidents or disease (e.g., cancer), who require reconstruction of facial features and tissues beyond the oral cavity; also orthognathic surgery.

- **Oral pathology** – the field of diagnosis and treatment of oral disease that may affect the entire body. The **oral pathologist** is a dental specialist who studies diseases and conducts research related to the oral cavity and diseases.

- **Orthodontics** – the field of correction of dental deformities and **anomalies** through the adjustment, alignment, and movement of teeth and their supporting structures. An **orthodontist** is a dental specialist who applies dental braces, fashions retainers, and other appliances to straighten the teeth and align jaw movements for chewing function and **esthetics.**

- **Endodontics** – the field of diagnosis, cause, prevention, and treatment of diseases of the dental pulp and related tissues. An **endodontist** is a dental specialist who performs root canals and related procedures, such as *apicoectomies* and *retrograde amalgams*.

- **Pediatric dentistry** (formerly referred to as *pedodontics*) – the field of treatment of children's teeth. A **pediatric dentist** (formerly called a *pedodontist)* is a dental specialist who treats children from their first dental visit through approximately age 18.
- **Public health dentistry** – the field of study, prevention, and treatment of dental diseases through community, county, state, and federal programs and agencies. A **public health dentist** is a dental specialist who provides dental services to a variety of population groups under the sponsorship of these agencies or programs.

The Dental Hygienist

The **dental hygienist** is a member of the dental health team whose duties include the prevention of oral diseases and the preservation of the natural teeth. The dental hygienist performs **oral prophylaxis** (tooth cleaning, deep scaling, and curettage) procedures for patients and applies decay-preventing agents such as *topical fluoride* and *pit and fissure sealants.*

The dental hygienist also polishes tooth surfaces and removes stains, dental plaque, and calculus (tartar). The dental hygienist exposes oral radiographs and provides nutritional and preventive oral hygiene instruction and counseling to patients.

The dental hygienist works under *general* or *direct* supervision of the dentist and may have a chairside assistant (see *Chapter 2, Legal and Ethical Issues and Responsibilities* for additional information on supervision).

The requirements for becoming a dental hygienist include a high school diploma or equivalent, and an associate's degree in dental hygiene from a program accredited by the *Commission on Dental Education of the American Dental Association.* Many hygienists also earn a bachelor of science degree.

The dental hygienist must pass a written national board and a written and clinical state board examination to be *licensed* in the state of employment. (*Note:* Practicing dental hygiene without a license is subject to disciplinary action by the State Board of Dental Examiners.) Upon satisfactory completion of the testing and licensing requirements, the hygienist becomes an *RDH* (Registered Dental Hygienist) in most states or an *LDH* (Licensed Dental Hygienist). The hygienist must follow all rules, regulations, and statutes set forth by the *State Dental Practice Act.*

Upon satisfactory completion of additional courses or expanded duties training, the dental hygienist may also perform *expanded functions*, such as administration of local anesthesia, placing and removing sutures, and placing and carving of permanent dental restorations. Note that these expanded duties must be performed under the direct supervision of the dentist or as outlined by the individual State Dental Practice Act.

The two recognized national professional associations for hygienists are the *American Dental Hygienists' Association* (ADHA) and the *National Dental Hygienists Association* (NDHA). Most dental hygienists also belong to their state dental hygiene association, through which they take continuing education courses as required for licensure renewal.

The Dental Office Manager

The **dental office manager** is in charge of all business aspects associated with running the practice. Depending upon the size of the office, she or he may also act as receptionist, appointment secretary, and billing clerk. In larger practices, the office manager may supervise a number of business (front office) and chairside (clinical) personnel.

Many office managers are former chairside dental assistants familiar with the clinical aspects of the practice, as well as terminology, supply inventory and control, and the personnel requirements of the dentist.

The dental office manager may be on-the-job trained, or may have had formal training as a dental assistant. The office manager may be certified, licensed, or registered, or possess a combination of these credentials. The office manager may have a business background or business major degree.

The two national professional organizations for all dental assistants, including office managers and chairside dental assistants, are the *American Dental Assistants Association* (ADAA) and the *National Association of Dental Assistants* (NADA). Many dental office managers and chairside assistants belong to state and local chapters, which are a source of continuing education courses required for credential renewal (Figure 1-1).

The Chairside Dental Assistant

The **chairside dental assistant** works in the **operatory** or treatment room with the dentist. The chairside assistant may be on-the-job trained or may

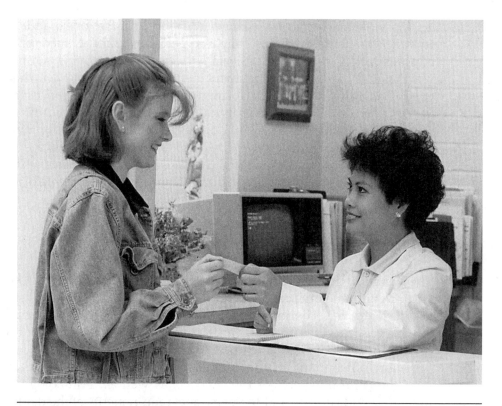

Figure 1-1. The office manager handles dental office business procedures. *(reprinted courtesy Registered Dental Assisting Program, Pasadena City College, Pasadena, CA.)*

have had formal training. The chairside assistant may be *licensed, registered,* or *certified,* or possess a combination of these credentials, or be on-the-job trained. With additional training, the chairside assistant may also be credentialed in expanded functions, as permitted by the state of employment.

The chairside assistant mixes and prepares dental impression and restorative materials, evacuates debris and extraneous materials from the oral cavity, and prepares the operatory for procedures including instrument tray and anesthesia set-ups as required by the dentist.

The chairside assistant exposes, processes, and mounts dental radiographs (x-rays) and may be required to hold a radiography license or certificate in the state of employment.

The chairside assistant may also perform dental instrument sterilization duties and prepare cases to be sent to an outside dental laboratory. The assistant may perform some dental laboratory procedures within the office, and is often the person responsible for infection control and sterilization requirements as set forth in government regulations and guidelines.

The chairside dental assistant works under *general* or *direct supervision* of the dentist (see *Chapter 2, Legal and Ethical Issues and Responsibilities* for further information) and is legally allowed to perform *only* those duties outlined by the State Dental Practice Act in the state of employment. With additional training, the chairside assistant may become an expanded duties assistant (Figure 1-2).

The Dental Laboratory Technician

The **dental laboratory technician** is also a member of the dental team. The dental laboratory technician may be on-the-job trained or may be formally trained and certified. *CDT* stands for Certified Dental Technician.

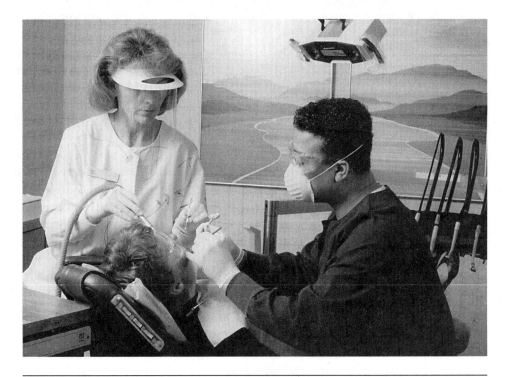

Figure 1-2. The dentist and dental assistant work as a team to provide quality dental care for the patient.

The dental laboratory technician fabricates dental prostheses such as crowns, bridges, and dentures, and orthodontic appliances such as retainers and tooth-bleaching trays, on the written direction or prescription of the dentist. The dental laboratory technician is *not* required to work under the supervision of the dentist, but may be required to adhere to regulations set forth in the State Dental Practice Act.

Many larger practices employ a dental laboratory technician in the office. However, most technicians work in an independent laboratory separate from the dental practice and provide laboratory services for numerous dental offices.

The Denturist

The **denturist** is *not* officially recognized by the American Dental Association. However, some states issue licenses to practice denturism. A denturist takes impressions of the oral cavity and fashions full and partial dentures for patients.

In some states the denturist must work under the supervision of a licensed dentist and must have completed the educational requirements outlined by the State Dental Practice Act to meet licensure requirements.

The Infection Control Coordinator

The role of **infection control coordinator** may be any member of the dental team to whom these duties are assigned, in addition to existing duties. This designated staff member is in charge of ensuring that sound infection control and sterilization techniques are conducted and documented, as required by government guidelines. There are no specific educational requirements for an infection coordinator at this time. However, certification in infection control is available through the **Dental Assisting National Board (DANB).**

Additional Personnel

Although not directly employed in the dental office, other dental professionals may have frequent contact with the dentist and staff.

The **dental supply representative** may call on the office in person or may have contact via the telephone. The dental supply representative provides products and services, including dental products, stationery items, and automatic inventory maintenance and shipment. The dental supply representative is also a source of information on new products, special pricing, and methods to make the practice more efficient.

The **dental service representative** may be called to perform routine maintenance and repair service work on dental equipment. The dental service representative also installs new dental equipment.

Qualifications and Credentials of the Dental Assistant

As stated previously, the dental office manager or chairside dental assistant may be trained on the job or may have received formal training. The following are credentials that may be earned by the dental office manager and chairside dental assistant.

Licensure and Registration

A number of states have licensure and registration provisions for dental assistants. These regulations may include successful completion of a formal training program, radiography proficiency, and a written or clinical examination. Some states accept completion of the Dental Assisting National Board (DANB) examination as a criterion for granting registration. Many states require periodic renewal of licensure or registration.

To obtain specific information regarding licensure and registration by state, the office manager may contact the American Dental Association Survey Center for a copy of *Legal Provisions for Delegation of Functions to Dental Hygienists and Dental Assistants*. Also, the office manager may contact her or his State Board of Dental Examiners for further information regarding licensure and registration requirements.

Certification

Certification may be earned in one of several areas. Upon successful completion of the requirements set forth by DANB, the dental office manager or chairside dental assistant may use the credential **"Certified Dental Assistant" (CDA)** following her or his name and may wear the DANB pin.

DANB has established respective designations of certification with specific eligibility *pathways* for each. They include: *Certified Dental Assistant (CDA), Certified Orthodontic Assistant (COA), Certified Oral and Maxillofacial Surgery Assistant (COMSA),* and *Certified Dental Practice Management Assistant (CDPMA).*

Those desiring certification must meet one of the eligibility *pathways* and must pass the examination related to the area of certification desired. Each pathway requires proof of current cardiopulmonary resuscitation (CPR) certification from either the American Heart Association or the American Red Cross.

Eligibility Pathways for Certification

The following are eligibility pathways by which the dental assistant may become certified.

Certified Dental Assistant (CDA)

The CDA exam includes three components: general chairside duties, infection control (ICE), and radiation health and safety (RHS). The three pathways to become a Certified Dental Assistant (CDA) are:

Pathway I:

- graduation from a dental assisting program or dental hygiene program accredited by the Commission on Dental Accreditation of the American Dental Association
- current CPR Healthcare Provider Level certification as prescribed by the American Heart Association or the American Red Cross

Pathway II:

- high school graduation or equivalent; and
- a minimum of two years of full-time work experience (3,500 hours) as a dental assistant verified by the dentist-employer; and
- current CPR Healthcare Provider Level certification as prescribed by the American Heart Association or the American Red Cross

Pathway III:

- previous DANB CDA certification with a lapsed status of three months or more and not meeting eligibility requirements for the CDA Reinstatement examination; and
- current CPR Healthcare Provider Level certification as prescribed by the American Heart Association or the American Red Cross

Certified Orthodontic Assistant (COA)

The COA examination consists of two components: infection control (ICE) and orthodontic assisting. The four pathways to become a Certified Orthodontic Assistant (COA) are:

Pathway I:

- work experience in an orthodontic practice setting and a CDA, RDH, or RDA credential; and
- current CPR Healthcare Provider Level certification as prescribed by the American Heart Association or the American Red Cross

Pathway II:

- high school graduation or equivalent; and
- a minimum of two years' full-time work experience (at least 3,500 hours) as an orthodontic assistant, verified by a dentist-employer; and
- current CPR Healthcare Provider Level certification as prescribed by the American Heart Association or the American Red Cross

Pathway III:

- completion of an orthodontic assisting preparation course at an institution having a dental assisting program accredited by the Commission on Dental Accreditation of the American Dental Association, plus the CDA credential; and
- current CPR Healthcare Provider Level certification as prescribed by the American Heart Association or the American Red Cross

Pathway IV:

- previous DANB COA certification with a lapsed status of three months or more; and

- current CPR Healthcare Provider Level certification as prescribed by the American Heart Association or the American Red Cross

Certified Oral and Maxillofacial Surgery Assistant (COMSA)

The COMSA exam includes two components: infection control (ICE) and oral and maxillofacial surgery assisting (OMS). The four pathways to become a Certified Oral and Maxillofacial Surgery Assistant (COMSA) are:

Pathway I:

- high school graduation or equivalent; and
- successful completion of 500 hours of post-secondary education in oral and maxillofacial surgery assisting; plus six months of full-time work experience (875 hours) in an oral and maxillofacial surgery practice setting or the equivalent; and
- current CPR Healthcare Provider Level certification as prescribed by the American Heart Association or the American Red Cross

Pathway II:

- work experience in an oral and maxillofacial surgery practice setting, plus a CDA, LPN, RN, RDH, or RDA credential; and
- current CPR Healthcare Provider Level certification as prescribed by the American Heart Association or the American Red Cross

Pathway III:

- high school graduation or equivalent; and
- a minimum of two years' full-time work experience (at least 3,500 hours) as an OMS assistant, verified by the dentist-employer; and
- current CPR Healthcare Provider Level certification as prescribed by the American Heart Association or the American Red Cross

Pathway IV:

- previous DANB COMSA certification with a lapsed status of three months or more; and
- current CPR Healthcare Provider Level certification as prescribed by the American Heart Association or the American Red Cross

Certified Dental Practice Management Assistant (CDPMA)

The CDPMA exam includes 200 multiple choice items. Dental radiography and infection control questions are included, but are not scored as separate components. The three pathways to become a Certified Dental Practice Management Assistant (CDPMA) are:

Pathway I:

- high school graduation or equivalent; and
- work experience in a dental practice setting verified by the dentist-employer; and
- current CPR Healthcare Provider Level certification as prescribed by the American Heart Association or the American Red Cross

Pathway II:

- high school graduation or equivalent; and
- completion of a practice management course at an institution having a dental assisting program accredited by the American Dental Association's Commission on Dental Accreditation; and
- current CPR Healthcare Provider Level certification as prescribed by the American Heart Association or the American Red Cross

Pathway III:

- previous DANB CDPMA certification with a lapsed status of three months or more; and
- current CPR Healthcare Provider Level certification as prescribed by the American Heart Association or the American Red Cross

The infection control exam (ICE) and dental radiation health and safety exam (RHS) may be taken by any individual without prerequisites. DANB does *not* set eligibility requirements for taking these exams. However, some states may require various eligibility standards because successful completion of these tests may complete that state's requirements for certification. As stated previously, the ICE and RHS exams comprise two-thirds of the CDA exam. (The remaining one-third covers general chairside questions.)

Additional information about certification testing requirements and dates may be obtained by contacting the Dental Assisting National Board in Chicago at (800) 367-3262.

Continuing Education

Education is a lifelong process. The dental office manager and chairside dental assistant are encouraged to participate in their career enrichment by taking advantage of continuing education courses offered through state, regional, and national dental organizations. Continuing education enhances self-esteem, upgrades and improves existing skills, and provides an opportunity for advancement within the practice.

Recertification Guidelines

Certified Dental Assistants must take a minimum of 12 hours of accredited continuing dental education (CDE) courses annually to renew certification. There are nine sources from which *certificants* may obtain continuing dental education credits:

1. *On-site lectures, courses, seminars, table clinics, and exhibits* – The CDA may earn one hour of continuing dental education credit for each clock hour of attendance at dental, dental hygiene, or dental assisting meetings sponsored by recognized dental groups.

   One hour maximum is awarded for one hour's time reviewing exhibits at dental meetings.

2. *Home study courses* – The CDA may successfully complete home study courses preapproved by the Dental Assisting National Board (DANB).

3. *Reading* – The CDA may earn a maximum of one CDE credit annually by reading. The certificant must maintain a log that demonstrates ongoing efforts to keep current with advances in dentistry through review of current literature. The log must include the title, author, date of publication, and name of the publication.

4. *Community participation* – The CDA may earn a maximum of one CDE hour annually by participating in community service, such as voluntary clinic work or speaking to students or other groups on dental health. The volunteer time must be a minimum of two hours to earn one credit.

5. *College courses* – The CDA may earn 12 CDE hours for *each* college course successfully completed. College courses must be related directly to dentistry or dental assisting.

6. *Taking DANB exams* – The CDA may earn 12 CDE credits for successful completion of a DANB-administered examination, *excluding* the initial certification exam. The CDA may take any of the following: RHS, ICE, CDA, COMSA, COA, CDPMA, or any DANB state-contracted exam.

7. *Cardiopulmonary (CPR) courses* – The CDA may earn a maximum of four CDE hours annually for successful completion of a CPR Health Care Provider Level course sponsored by the American Heart Association or the American Red Cross.

8. *Scholarly activity* – The CDA may earn a maximum of three CDE hours annually by participating in any of the following activities:
   - present a continuing dental education program
   - write a published article in the dental field
   - teach a professional course directly related to dentistry or dental assisting
   - serve on a DANB test construction committee
   - submit six DANB exam items accepted by the DANB committee

9. *Electives* – The CDA may earn a maximum of three CDE hours annually for attending a professional development course directly related to the delivery of patient services such as stress management, staff motivation, or team building (Figure 1-3).

Continuing Education Audit

All CDAs are subject to a random continuing dental education (CDE) audit at annual renewal. Those randomly selected for CDE verification

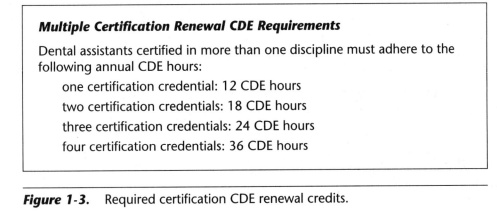

Multiple Certification Renewal CDE Requirements

Dental assistants certified in more than one discipline must adhere to the following annual CDE hours:

    one certification credential: 12 CDE hours

    two certification credentials: 18 CDE hours

    three certification credentials: 24 CDE hours

    four certification credentials: 36 CDE hours

Figure 1-3.   Required certification CDE renewal credits.

must provide proof of continuing education. Proof of completed continuing education should be retained for two years in the event of subsequent audit. Certificants not selected for audit will have their certification renewal for one full year. However, proof of CDE should be retained for the previous two years.

Working Together as a Team

It is imperative that all members of the dental team work together to provide the best care and service possible to patients. In addition to effective communication techniques and treating each other with respect, it is vital that the team routinely address issues that affect the practice. Some issues may be addressed and solutions reached as they arise. Others require additional discussion and planning and are best handled through staff meetings.

Staff Meetings

Staff meetings, sometimes referred to as team meetings, are held on a routine basis with all employees of the practice attending and participating. These guidelines help ensure the office manager organizes effective staff meetings:

- Block out the meeting time in the appointment schedule. Meetings should be scheduled at the same times (the same weekly or monthly time, for example), at regular intervals.
- Prepare an agenda with specific time blocks to ensure the team stays on schedule and stays focused on the topics to be addressed. Planning the meeting with the dentist, it is the office manager's responsibility to see that the topics the dentist wants covered are on the meeting agenda.
- Start staff meetings on time and finish on time.
- Take responsibility for facilitating (running) the staff meeting to ensure everyone on staff has experience as a facilitator.
- Assign a recorder to take notes and provide a written action plan resulting from the meeting.

- Provide a large newsprint pad, flip chart, or writing board to record brainstorming sessions and action ideas.

Although staff members run the meeting, the dentist has the following responsibilities:

- to cast a deciding or final vote when the team is divided on an issue or where significant financial considerations apply
- to aid the facilitator in keeping the meeting on time and focused as necessary
- to introduce significant changes in the practice
- to review progress of action items with each staff member, if necessary, and then lead the team with follow-up and recognition (Figure 1-4)

The Morning Huddle

The morning huddle is a brief meeting at the beginning of the day to set the tone, strategize procedures, and discuss patients' specific needs. It is the office manager's job to provide information to the dentist for the

Team Meeting Action Plan				
Goal	Person Responsible	Action Required	By Date	Result/ Outcome

Figure 1-4. Sample team-meeting action plan.

morning huddle to enhance communication and cooperation between business and clinical staff, to provide improved patient service, and to increase the overall productivity of the practice.

The morning huddle may include the following:

- *Specific concerns from the previous day* – How could the schedule have run more smoothly? How were cancellations or disappointments handled? What could be done better next time to avoid these?

- *Highlight today's schedule* – Who are the new patients? Are there openings in the schedule and how will they be filled? Is the call list up to date?

- *Emergency and catch-up time* – Are there any flexible times where additional treatment could be accomplished? How much time is available?

- *Preblocked production times* – Are all the crucial production times blocked? When is the next available time open?

- *Financial information about the patients booked today* – Are insurance claims filed for predetermination? Are there any accounts overdue? Have financial arrangements been confirmed before proceeding with initial restorative treatment?

- *Marketing opportunities* – Is the tracking sheet for new patients up to date? What are the sources of new patients? What is the practice doing to gain new patients? How is the practice thanking those who refer new patients?

Goal Setting

One of the important elements that arises from staff meetings is goal setting. The **practice goals** are an extension of the practice philosophy and mission statement. They are broken down into measurable results, such as quality and promptness of service, number of surfaces restored, percentage of recall patients rescheduled, number of new patients scheduled, promptness of seating patients, or answering the telephone.

The practice's productivity, and ultimately the staff's rewards, come partly as a result of meeting practice goals, including production goals.

Quality Assurance

Establishing standards for the highest-quality dental care is another essential that arises from staff meetings and goal setting. Quality to the dentist is equated with outstanding technical skill; quality to the patient is a perception that includes outstanding communication, satisfaction, and being treated with courtesy and respect by the dentist and staff. In reality, *quality is a judgment that includes both technical skills and the management of communication exchanges between the patient and the practice.*

Continuous quality improvement and *total quality management* emphasize continuous improvement through understanding and knowledge about the processes (procedures) and techniques used to provide care, the health results achieved, and an emphasis on the patients' perceived needs and demands. This customer service philosophy reflects patients' involvement in their care and obtaining the necessary information they need to make informed decisions about their dental health (Figure 1-5).

Patient Perceptions That Determine Quality of Care

- **How dental conditions affect daily function and well-being.** If a patient has an abscessed tooth and fever, how will he or she perform at his or her job today?

- **Treatment needs.** If this patient is diagnosed as requiring a root canal, how will the dental team provide this care?

- **Satisfaction with the process (procedure) of care.** How satisfied is the patient with elements of service, e.g., how soon was his or her telephone call answered? How quickly was he or she appointed? Was pain medication administered appropriately? Was he or she treated with courtesy and compassion by the dentist and staff? Were all his or her questions answered to his or her satisfaction?

- **Treatment efficacy.** Did the root canal treatment relieve his or her pain and pressure? Did the prescribed medications control the symptoms? Did the final result meet or exceed his or her expectations?

Figure 1-5. Patient perceptions that determine quality of care.

Skill-Building for Success: Student Activities

These optional activities and exercises are designed to help the student put into practice information learned in the chapter.

1. Divide into groups or work on your own, and take approximately 10 minutes to develop a sample practice philosophy or mission statement. At the completion, share your philosophy or mission statement with the class. Give positive input and discuss the results.

2. List the eight recognized dental specialties. Describe what each of these dental specialists does.

3. Make a list of all the team members who work in a dental office. List the educational requirements and job descriptions for each.

4. List the types of formal credentials available to the dental office manager and chairside dental assistant and the requirements for each. List the pathways for certification eligibility.

5. List sources of continuing education for the dental office manager and chairside dental assistant and describe why continuing education is important.

6. Role play a staff meeting or morning huddle, using fictitious names to describe situations and how they can be resolved. Possible concerns may include: a) a patient is scheduled for a crown and bridge appointment and has not made financial arrangements; b) a patient of record calls with a toothache and demands to be seen today; c) monthly statements are not getting out on time.

7. Describe what quality of care is as perceived by the dentist, the patient, and the staff.

Skills Mastery Assessment: Post-Test

Directions: Select the response that best answers each of the following questions. Only one response is correct.

1. To ensure a well-run office, the dental office manager must be familiar with the practice's:
   a. philosophy and mission statement
   b. goals
   c. a and b only
   d. all of the above

2. The first priority of the dental team is to:
   a. collect all outstanding accounts receivable
   b. serve all patients with courtesy and a quality, service-oriented philosophy
   c. set up staff meetings
   d. define total quality management

3. To work in private practice the dentist must be:
   a. a graduate of a dental school approved by the Commission on Dental Accreditation of the American Dental Association
   b. licensed in the state of employment
   c. a member of the State Board of Dental Examiners
   d. a and b only

4. A dental specialist may practice within any scope of dental treatment, including one or more of the eight recognized specialties.
   a. True
   b. False
   c. there are only six recognized dental specialties

5. A periodontist performs:
   a. gingival (gum) treatments
   b. root canals
   c. fixed prosthetics
   d. all of the above

6. An oral surgeon is a dental specialist who:
   a. extracts teeth
   b. exposes impacted teeth
   c. wires fractured jaws
   d. all of the above

7. The dental hygienist:
   a. performs oral prophylaxis (tooth cleaning) procedures
   b. applies decay-preventing agents
   c. exposes oral radiographs
   d. all of the above

8. The dental hygienist works under *general* or *direct* supervision of the dentist and may work with a chairside assistant.
   a. True
   b. False

9. The dental office manager:
   a. is in charge of all business aspects associated with running the practice
   b. may act as receptionist, appointment secretary, and billing clerk
   c. may supervise a number of business (front office) and chairside (clinical) assistants in a larger practice
   d. any / all of the above

10. The chairside dental assistant:
    a. performs deep scaling and curettage procedures
    b. is required to be licensed in the state of employment
    c. mixes and prepares dental impression and restorative materials
    d. may use the initials RDH after his or her name

11. The chairside dental assistant:
    a. prepares the operatory for procedures
    b. prepares instrument trays and anesthesia set-ups as required by the dentist
    c. performs dental instrument sterilization duties as set forth by government regulations and guidelines
    d. all of the above

12. The dental laboratory technician:
    a. fabricates dental prostheses
    b. makes orthodontic appliances
    c. is required to work under the supervision of the dentist
    d. a and b only

13. Licensure and registration for dental assistants are regulated by the individual state in which the assistant is employed.
    a. True
    b. False

14. Designations for certification granted by the Dental Assisting National Board include:
    a. Certified Dental Assistant (CDA)
    b. Certified Oral and Maxillofacial Surgery Assistant (COMSA)
    c. Certified Dental Practice Management Assistant (CDPMA)
    d. all of the above are designated certification areas

15. Dental office managers or chairside assistants wishing to become certified through the Dental Assisting National Board must meet all pathway requirements and pass the examination related to the area of certification desired.
    a. True
    b. False

16. Each certification pathway requires proof of current cardiopulmonary resuscitation (CPR) certification from either the American Heart Association or the American Red Cross.
    a. True
    b. False

17. The CDA may earn continuing education credits by:
    a. attending on-site dental lectures, courses, seminars, table clinics, and exhibits
    b. taking preapproved home study courses
    c. taking DANB-administered examinations
    d. all of the above

18. The office manager can organize effective staff meetings by:
    a. blocking out the meeting time in the appointment schedule
    b. preparing an agenda to ensure the team stays on schedule and stays focused
    c. assigning a recorder to take notes and provide a written action plan resulting from the meeting
    d. all of the above

19. The morning huddle may include:
    a. specific concerns from the previous day
    b. emergency and catch-up time
    c. financial information about patients booked
    d. all of the above

20. Quality is a judgment that includes both technical skills and the management of communication exchanges between the patient and the practice.
    a. True
    b. False

References

1998 Recertification Guidelines. (1997, November). *The Certified Press.* Chicago: Dental Assisting National Board.

Certified dental assistant examination fact sheets. Chicago: Dental Assisting National Board.

Pride, J. (1997, December). A time to share good ideas. *Dental Economics.*

Stewart, D. (1996, Fall). Quality in oral health care. *Preview.*

Tucci, D. (1996, January/February). Expanding staff roles by delegating. *Journal of the American Dental Assistants Association/The Dental Assistant.*

Chapter 2

Legal and Ethical Issues and Responsibilities

- **Dental Jurisprudence**
- **Dental Ethics**
- **The State Board of Dental Examiners**
- **Code of Ethics**
  - The ADA Code of Ethics
  - The ADAA Code of Ethics
- **Supervision of Staff**
  - General Supervision
  - Direct Supervision
- **Personnel Policies**
- **The Importance of an Office Manual**
- **Hiring Issues**
  - Fair Hiring Practices
  - Quality of Work Environment
  - Harassment
  - Employee Behavior
  - Written Job Descriptions
  - Provisional Employment
  - Employee Leasing and Temporary Employment Services
  - Performance Reviews
  - Termination
  - Wrongful Discharge
- **Employee Salary and Benefits**
  - Paid Leave

Unpaid Leave
Additional Benefits
- **Employee Records**
- **The Americans with Disabilities Act (AwDA)**
    Implications for the Dental Office
    Necessary Office Renovations
- **Risk Management Strategies to Prevent Malpractice**
    Negligence
    Standard of Care
    Abandonment
    Burden of Proof
    Elements of Malpractice
    Causes of Malpractice Suits
    Steps to Prevent Malpractice
    When an Accident Happens or a Patient Complains
- **When a Patient Declines or Discontinues Treatment**
- **Patient Confidentiality**
    Patient Confidentiality and the Fax Machine
- **Reporting Suspected Domestic Abuse**
    Signs and Symptoms of Domestic Abuse
    Child Abuse
    Spousal Abuse
    Reporting and Documenting Procedures

Learning Objectives

Upon completion of this chapter, the student will achieve an 80 percent or higher score on the Skills Mastery Assessment Post-Test *covering the following material.*

1. Define and describe the terms ethics and jurisprudence.

2. List the duties of the State Board of Dental Examiners.

3. Be familiar with the content and implications of the *American Dental Assistants Association Principles of Ethics and Professional Conduct.*

4. Define and describe the difference between general and direct supervision as they relate to the dental assistant.

5. Describe legal and financial aspects and hiring practices associated with employment in the dental office.

6. Describe the provisions and implications of the *Americans with Disabilities Act (AwDA)* as it pertains to the dental office.

7. Describe the importance of risk management in preventing dental malpractice.

8. Describe the legal requirements of dental offices to report suspected cases of domestic abuse.

Key Terms

abandonment

active abuse

Americans with Disabilities Act (AwDA)

benefits

burden of proof

child abuse

code of ethics

compensation

direct supervision

Equal Employment Opportunity Commission

ethics

general supervision

handicapped

impairment

informed consent

job description

jurisprudence

liable/liability

licensee

malpractice

National Practitioner Data Bank

negligence

noncompliance

overtime pay

paid leave

passive abuse

performance review

prognoses

provisional employment

proximate cause

risk management

severance pay

spousal abuse

standard of care

State Board of Dental Examiners

State Dental Practice Act

termination

unpaid leave

unprofessional conduct

Dental Jurisprudence

Dental **jurisprudence** is the application of legal statutes and other regulations that pertain to the *State Dental Practice Act.* Jurisprudence is a philosophy of law or a set of legal regulations set forth by each state's legislature.

By law, dental **licensees** must understand the obligations and privileges granted by the license; they must follow these rules and be aware of dental duties legally allowable in the state in which they practice.

Dental Ethics

Ethics is a moral obligation that encompasses professional conduct and judgment imposed by the members of a particular profession. The ethical standards are developed by the professional organization; those who participate in the profession are morally obligated to act within an ethical or moral manner. Ethics is considered a higher standard (moral) than jurisprudence (legal) requirements.

The State Board of Dental Examiners

Each state has a separate **Board of Dental Examiners,** empowered by the legislature to enforce the **State Dental Practice Act** to protect the health, safety, and welfare of the people residing in the particular state. The state board also regulates the criteria for dental licensees within the state, and issues and renews licenses for dental personnel practicing within the state. It monitors licensees and enforces discipline for **noncompliance.**

In states where registration of dental assistants is recognized, the state board may also regulate the criteria for assistants—including maintaining continuing educational standards and other requirements, such as radiology credentialing.

In states where expanded functions are permitted, the state regulates and enforces the limit and scope of allowable duties for assistants and hygienists. Working beyond the scope of the Dental Practice Act may be considered practicing dentistry without a license and is a serious offense.

Code of Ethics

A professional **code of ethics** is that which stands above the legal requirements of the dental profession.

The ADA Code of Ethics

The American Dental Association has developed and published the *Principles of Dental Ethics and Code of Professional Conduct*, to which all practicing dentists are morally obligated to adhere.

The ADAA Code of Ethics

The American Dental Assistants Association has also developed a set of *Principles of Ethics and Professional Conduct*, the standard by which all dental assistants, including clinical and managerial personnel, are expected to work (Figure 2-1).

American Dental Assistants Association
Principles of Ethics and Professional Conduct

Each individual involved in the practice of dentistry assumes the obligation of maintaining and enriching the profession. Each member shall choose to meet this obligation according to the dictates of personal conscience based on the needs of the general public the profession of dentistry is committed to serve.

The member shall refrain from performing any professional service which is prohibited by state law, and has the obligation to prove competence prior to providing services to any patient. The member shall constantly strive to upgrade and expand technical skills for the benefit of the employer and consumer public. This member should additionally seek to sustain and improve the local organization, state association, and the American Dental Assistants Association through active participation and personal commitment.

Figure 2-1. "American Dental Assistants Association Principles of Ethics and Professional Conduct." *(reprinted with permission of the ADAA.)*

Supervision of Staff

By law, the dentist is responsible for all acts committed within the practice. This includes delegation of duties to properly trained personnel. Supervision of staff may be **general** or **direct**.

General Supervision

General supervision, in most states, means the dentist is responsible for all acts delegated to and performed by staff (within the law) but that the act itself may be done while the dentist is not physically present in the office. Examples of a dental assistant's duties under general supervision are processing dental radiographs and sterilizing instruments.

The dentist is responsible for the diagnostic quality of the radiographs, but does not have to be in the office at the time of processing. Likewise, the dentist is legally responsible for meeting or exceeding the standards of instrument sterilization; however, she or he need not be in the office while the assistant processes instruments.

Direct Supervision

Direct supervision includes overseeing of specific delegatable duties, as stipulated in the State Dental Practice Act as allowable for trained staff to perform. The dentist *must* be present in the facility while these procedures are being performed. Examples of this are taking radiographs on patients or performing coronal polish procedures (where permitted by the individual State Dental Practice Act).

Personnel Policies

For optimal communication and to prevent misunderstandings, most offices have written guidelines in the form of a personnel policy manual. In most states (31) the courts have ruled personnel policies, procedures manuals, and employee handbooks may be legally binding (implied) contracts; of the remaining states, courts in five have ruled manuals and handbooks are *not* legally binding contracts.

The Importance of an Office Manual

Having a single source of written office policies and procedures is essential in preventing misunderstandings. It also provides a standard of fairness and consistency for all employees, especially in larger clinics or group practices. The office manual may be the "final word" when office policies are questioned.

An office manual is a reflection of the management style of the practice that outlines the practice philosophy, policies, procedures, and employee behavior guidelines.

All new dental personnel should be provided with a copy of the office manual when hired. Personnel of record are advised to review the manual at least once annually thereafter.

From time to time the office manual may be adapted or updated to reflect changes in employment laws or other government regulations, such as the wearing of personal protective equipment for disease containment. (See *Chapter 3, Hazard Communication and Other Regulatory Agency Mandates,* for further information.)

It is important to note that the office manual also provides protection for the employee in the event of exposure to a potentially hazardous substance or an accidental injury. Further, because of the volume of information and wide variety of procedures, some offices have several different manuals, which may cover personnel issues, hazard communication, and Material Safety Data Sheets, individually. (The latter two are also addressed in *Chapter 3.*)

Hiring Issues

A well-run office is one in which all staff and the dentist work together as a team to serve patients. A key to keeping the work flow productive is sound communication skills that build positive relationships within the office. This should be emphasized during the interview process and reinforced at staff meetings.

When hiring a new employee, consensus of the team is essential to ensure a successful training period and introduction to the practice's procedures and philosophy.

Fair Hiring Practices

Employers and prospective staff members must be aware of specific topics that may or may not be discussed during an interview for employment. These standards are set by the Federal Government through the **Equal Employment Opportunity Commission (EEOC)** under *Title VII* of the *Civil Rights Act* of 1964. They are designed to ensure all individuals the right to compete for employment opportunities, as well as to reduce the potential for hiring discrimination based upon a variety of factors. These include, but may not be limited to, questions regarding race, color, religion, sex, national origin, age, or disability.

The dentist as employer, by law, has the right to select whomever she or he believes is the best-qualified candidate to perform the responsibilities and duties of a specific job. Under current employment laws the employer is *not* required to select the *most qualified candidate;* he or she is only required to select a candidate who meets the *minimum requirements* of the job.

Quality of Work Environment

The dentist as employer must ensure that all state laws regarding quality of the work environment are upheld for the health, welfare, protection, and safety of all employees. Failure to uphold these codes may result in fines, penalties, or restriction of practice.

For example, the employer must also ensure that hazards such as poor ventilation, protection from radiation, and potential for accidents and injuries are minimized.

Harassment

The law contains specific wording on the nature and definition of harassment in the workplace. Simply defined, harassment consists of any unwanted or unwelcome advances by an employer or supervisor toward a subordinate employee, especially where continued employment, advancement, or favors are implicit or explicit based upon compliance. Many office manuals contain a copy of guidelines regarding harassment.

Employee Behavior

The office manual should outline specific expectations of employee behavior, including keeping office hours, policies on tardiness, and personal telephone usage.

Written Job Descriptions

To avoid misunderstandings and to clearly communicate the expectations of the employer, it is essential that a written **job description** be made available to the candidate. A copy of each staff member's job description should be included in the office manual and a copy should be provided to the candidate at the employment interview.

As job responsibilities change, the job description should also be updated. A printed, dated copy should be provided to the employee. At the time of the annual performance review, both the dentist-employer and the staff member should review the written job description (Figure 2-2) (Figure 2-3) (Figure 2-4).

Provisional Employment

After completing a successful applicant interview, the dentist may elect to hire a new staff member provisionally. **Provisional employment,** by written notice on office letterhead, outlines the starting date, the rate of compensation, the hours of service, and other benefits included with the position. The benefit of entering into provisional employment is that either the dentist or the staff member may, at any time during the provisional period (customarily 90 days), elect to discontinue the employment arrangement without prior notice and without cause (reason). Under provisional employment agreements, no unemployment benefits are awarded.

Employee Leasing and Temporary Employment Services

Many businesses today, including dental practices, engage outside agencies to provide leased employees. The advantages to the practice include prescreening of applicants, administration of payroll and benefits is han-

RECEPTIONIST/OFFICE MANAGER DUTIES

Name____

Date____

Routinely Perform	Occasionally Perform	Never Perform	Duties	Trainee	Assistant	Senior Receptionist	Principal Receptionist
			1. Schedules new patients for appointments to see.	Procedure Training	Procedure Competency	Procedure Competency	Procedure Competency
			2. Schedules patients (both new and recall) to see the Dental Hygienist.				
			3. Maintains patient records.				
			4. Develops and maintains an effective recall system for patients who have completed treatment.				
			5. Develops and maintains effective inventory control of recyclable, consumable and expendable supplies.				
			6. Orders all supplies for clinical and business office use.				
			7. Discusses financial arrangements with patients.		Training		
			8. Arranges payment schedule for patients receiving treatment.				
			9. Submits statements monthly to all patients with account balances.				
			10. Maintains patient accounts to minimize delinquent accounts.				
			11. Collects fees from patients.				
			12. Maintains business records of the practice.			Training	
			13. Submits payment for office expenses.				
			14. Reconciles check book with bank statement monthly.				
			15. Cooperates with other professional and auxiliary staff.				

Minimal Desirable Qualifications

1. High school graduation.
2. Ability to work in a semi-autonomous manner.
3. Good secretarial skills.
4. Bookkeeping skills.

Work Schedule

The normal work schedule for this individual will be eight hours per day five days each week for a total of 40 hours per week.

It is expected that this individual will work 50 weeks per year, with two weeks paid vacation after the first full year of employment. There will be five to eight paid holidays per year.

Salary

1. Annual Salary of____________.
2. __________% of all office gross above____________.

Figure 2-2. Sample job description: dental receptionist/office manager. *(Reprinted courtesy of Drs. Thomas M. Cooper and John A. DiBiaggio from* Applied Practice Management.*)*

DENTAL ASSISTANT DUTIES

Name _____

Date _____

Routinely Perform	Occasionally Perform	Never Perform	Duties	Trainee	Assistant	Senior Assistant	Principal Assistant
			1. Perform basic administrative office procedures.	Procedure Training	Procedure Competency	Procedure Competency	Procedure Competency
			2. Assist the dentist in four-handed dentistry.				
			3. Prepare tray setups for commonly performed procedures.				
			4. Record oral examinations as directed by the dentist.				
			5. Prepare and clean instruments.				
			6. Prepare and sterilize instruments.				
			7. Pour and trim diagnostic models.				
			8. Construct custom acrylic trays.				
			9. Assist in administration of local anesthetics.				
			10. Prepare dental materials as indicated for treatment.				
			11. Assist with placement and removal of rubber dam.				
			12. Assist with placement of bases and liners.				
			13. Assist in insertion and finishing of temporary restorations.				
			14. Assist in insertion and finishing of composite restorations.				
			15. Assist in placement and removal of matrices.				
			16. Assist in insertion and carving of amalgam restorations.				
			17. Assist with first aid and emergency procedures.	Training			
			18. Aid in the presentation of post-operative instructions.				
			19. Expose, process and mount radiographs.				
			20. Assist with advanced dental procedures.				
			21. Instruct other auxiliaries in dental assisting.			Training	
			22. Conduct demonstrations in assisting.				
			23. Evaluate new personnel for the purpose of grading.				
			24. Conduct ongoing in-service training for auxiliaries.				

Minimal Desirable Qualifications
1. High school graduation
2. Three years experience as dental assistant.

Work Schedule
The normal work schedule for this individual will be eight hours per day five days per week for a total of 40 hours per week.
It is expected that this individual will work 50 weeks per year, with two weeks paid vacation after the first full year of employment. There will be five to eight paid holidays per year.

Salary
1. Annual Salary of_____.
2. _____% of gross above_____.

Figure 2-3. Sample job description: dental assistant. *(Reprinted courtesy of Drs. Thomas M. Cooper and John A. DiBiaggio from Applied Practice Management.)*

DENTAL HYGIENIST DUTIES

Name____

Date____

Routinely Perform	Occasionally Perform	Never Perform		Assistant Dental Hyg.	Senior Hygienist	Principal Hygienist
			1. Promotes the maintenance of dental health among patients.	Pro. Competency	Procedure Competency	Procedure Competency
			2. Scales and polishes teeth.			
			3. Scales and planes root surfaces.			
			4. Topically applies caries preventive agents.			
			5. Desensitizes hypersensitive teeth and oral mucosa.			
			6. Maintains relative asepsis.			
			7. Removes overhanging margins.	Training		
			8. Removes and recements space maintainers.			
			9. Initiates or assists in administering emergency care for patients, and removes sutures and surgical packs from oral cavity.			
			10. Coordinates the office Preventive Dentistry Program.		Training	
			11. Designs and maintains an effective recall program.			
			12. Trains members of the dental team in preventive procedures.			

Minimal Desirable Qualifications

1. Graduation from a two-year accredited certificate program.
2. Must be licensed in this state.
3. Two years clinical experience.

Work Schedule

The normal work schedule for this individual will be eight hours per day five days each week for a total of 40 hours per week.

It is expected that this individual will work 50 weeks per year, with two weeks paid vacation after the first full year of employment. There will be five to eight paid holidays per year.

Salary

1. Annual Salary of__________.
2. ________% of all office gross above__________.

Figure 2-4. Sample job description: dental hygienist. *(Reprinted courtesy of Drs. Thomas M. Cooper and John A. DiBiaggio from* Applied Practice Management.*)*

dled outside the office, and the dentist has more time to devote to the practice. In large offices or clinics, it is the responsibility of the leasing firm to supply replacement employees to cover the office for vacation, sick days, and maternity leave.

Temporary employment services are used as a means of sourcing potential permanent employees. They are also used to cover vacation times, maternity leave, and extended leaves of absence.

Performance Reviews

Performance reviews, most often conducted annually, are essential to sustaining positive dentist-staff relationships. Performance reviews are based upon the objectives of performance expectation outlined in the individual staff member's written job description, along with a rating scale of performance of each duty.

The performance review should take place separately from the annual raise review to allow employees time to adjust to additional responsibilities and to focus on areas that require improvement. The office manager should note that the employer is *not* legally obligated to provide annual reviews or salary increases (Figure 2-5).

Termination

The terms of employment and **termination** should be outlined clearly in the office manual and should be explained to all new hires. This not only helps prevent misunderstandings, it reduces stress levels, eliminates anxiety, and creates a common understanding between employer and employee.

While the term *two weeks' notice* has been a standard of business practice for many years, it is a formal courtesy, and not governed by law. Thus, a staff member desiring to terminate her or his employment may give two weeks' written notice. However, the employer is *not* legally or ethically bound to continue her or his employment during this period.

Likewise, in the event the employer-dentist elects to terminate an employee, service may be terminated with little or no notice. Many employers, however, may choose to award **severance pay** based upon the length of service or to award unused vacation pay at termination. These terms should be outlined in the office manual.

PERFORMANCE REVIEW

NAME: DATE OF EMPLOYMENT:
STARTING SALARY: EXPERIENCE:

REVIEW DATE: EVALUATION AND COMMENTS:
SALARY CHANGE:

REVIEW DATE: EVALUATION AND COMMENTS:
SALARY CHANGE:

REVIEW DATE: EVALUATION AND COMMENTS:
SALARY CHANGE:

REVIEW DATE: EVALUATION AND COMMENTS:
SALARY CHANGE:

REVIEW DATE: EVALUATION AND COMMENTS:
SALARY CHANGE:

REVIEW DATE: EVALUATION AND COMMENTS:
SALARY CHANGE:

Figure 2-5. Sample performance review form. *(Reprinted   courtesy of Drs. Thomas M. Cooper and John A. DiBiaggio from* Applied Practice Management.*)*

Wrongful Discharge

Wrongful discharge (sometimes referred to as wrongful dismissal) stems from an employee alleging she or he was wrongfully terminated from employment. Grounds may include age discrimination, failure to comply with office policies, disputes arising from uncompensated overtime or vacation pay, or attitude. Whether pursued through the court system or through state employment commission grievance procedures, the onus is on the employee to prove beyond a reasonable doubt that the employer was guilty of wrongful discharge. This is often very difficult to prove.

Employee Salary and Benefits

Compensation to the employee is most often paid on an hourly rate or as weekly salary. **Overtime pay** is awarded to full-time hourly wage employees for working beyond the standard 40-hour work week.

In addition to hourly or weekly pay, **benefits,** usually provided only to full-time employees, represent a significant form of nontaxable compensation provided by the employer. Benefits may include paid vacation, sick days, compensation for reaching production goals, health insurance, or pension plan contributions.

Many employers provide quantitative information with the pay stub or annual wage and benefits statement that outlines the total value of the job, including employee benefits (Figure 2-6).

Paid Leave

Paid leave includes time away from the office taken for earned vacation, federal holidays, or sick time. Vacation pay or annual leave is customarily one or two weeks earned after one full year of satisfactory employment. With additional years of service, many employers provide an additional week's paid leave.

The six recognized paid federal holidays include, but may not be limited to, New Year's Day, Memorial Day, Independence Day, Labor Day, Thanksgiving, and Christmas. Some employers may also recognize bank holidays, including Martin Luther King Jr. Day, President's Day, Columbus Day, and Veteran's Day.

Paid sick time is awarded at the discretion of the employer. The specific terms should be outlined by the employer in the office manual.

Employee Name:			

Annual Employee Total Compensation/Cost

A. Direct Compensation	_ _ _ _ (estimate)	_ _ _ _ (actual)	_ _ _ _ (actual)
Gross Base Salary (Includes Vacation/Sick pay)			
Overtime (Pre-Tax Amount)			
Bonuses (Pre-Tax Amount)			
Employee Tax (Estimate 10% of Gross Salary)			
or FICA			
State Unemployment/FUTA			
Worker's Compensation Insurance			
*Retirement Plan Contribution (if 100% vested)			
Retirement Plan Administration Allocation			
B. Employee Fringe Benefits			
*Cafeteria Plan Reimbursement			
*Medical Insurance and Reimbursements			
*Group Life Insurance			
*Uniforms			
*Child Care ($5,000 Max)			
Tangible Awards Program (every 5 years)			
Annual Gift ($25 Max)			
Dental Care			
C. Career Benefits			
Dental Continuing Education			
Tuition and Travel Reimbursement			
Lodging and Meals			
Inoculations and OSHA Safety			
*Professional Dues & Subscriptions			
TOTAL COMPENSATION/COST			
D. Hidden Compensation			
Tax Savings (example for Illinois: FICA .07 + FED .28 + State .03 = 38% x all *)			
True per Hr. Wage (Total Compensation/Hrs.)			

Figure 2-6.   Employee compensation. *(Reprinted courtesy of Dental Economics.)*

Unpaid Leave

Many employers provide **unpaid leave,** that is, time away from the office for which the employee is not compensated. Unpaid leave may include maternity leave (after all sick leave and vacation days are exhausted), personal leave (for family emergencies), bereavement leave (for death of an immediate family member), or jury duty. The specific terms must be outlined by the employer in the office manual.

Additional Benefits

Other benefits not directly included in the paycheck but provided by the employer may include health and life insurance, retirement (pension plan) contributions, and uniform allowances. Many practices make these additional benefits available on a copayment basis to full-time employees, i.e., the employer and the employee share in the cost or contribution toward the benefit.

Some employers, especially those who require standard uniforms of matching clinic attire, award an annual uniform allowance toward the cost of these items. The terms of these additional benefits should also be outlined by the employer in the office manual.

Bonus or incentive programs may be offered to staff for exceptional performance on the job. Bonuses may be based upon goals set for numbers or percentages of increase in new patients, production, recall program retention, or collection of overdue accounts.

The cost of child or elder care may be an additional benefit shared by the employer and the employee.

Many employers also provide or share with staff the cost of additional skills training or continuing education. Examples include attendance at dental seminars, dental meetings, lodging and meals, paid subscriptions to dental periodicals, certification/registration/licensure renewal fees, and reduced fees for dental treatment for staff and their immediate family members. These benefits must also be outlined in the office manual.

By law, the cost of required inoculations (the hepatitis B vaccine) and OSHA safety regulations (personal protective equipment) is also absorbed by the employer (see *Chapter 3* for further information).

Employee Records

Accurate and thorough record keeping is the lifeline of the practice. Not only does this include patient clinical and accounting records, but also employee records. These records are confidential and include payroll, tax, disability, workers compensation, unemployment, and other information required by OSHA, including management of accidental injuries and work site accidents.

By law, dental offices are required to retain employee records for the duration of employment plus 30 years. In the event of the death of the doctor or sale of the practice, the records become the property of the new owner.

The Americans with Disabilities Act (AwDA)

Approximately 43 million Americans have some degree of disability. Enacted in 1992, the **Americans with Disabilities Act** (**AwDA**, also called the *Act*), applies specifically to dental offices, requiring facilities be accessible to handicapped (physically or mentally compromised) patients.

Implications for the Dental Office

The *Americans with Disabilities Act* enumerates five categories of persons who are protected from discrimination:

1. Persons with a physical or mental impairment that substantially limits one or more of the major life activities, such as seeing, hearing, speaking, walking, breathing, performing manual tasks, learning, caring for oneself, or working. Also included in this category are people who have disabling conditions, such as AIDS, HIV infections, heart disease, diabetes, cancer, learning disabilities, or mental retardation.

2. Persons who have a record of such an impairment, such as a history of cancer or a person with a history of mental illness.

3. Persons who, while fully functional and not actually disabled, are regarded as having such an impairment due to severe disfigurement.

4. Persons who are discriminated against because they have a known association or relationship with a disabled individual.

5. Persons who currently participate in or who have completed a drug or alcohol rehabilitation program.

Impairment, in general, means any physiological disorder or condition, cosmetic disfigurement, or anatomical loss. It can also mean any mental or psychological disorder, such as mental retardation, emotional or mental illness, or specific learning disabilities.

Handicapped patients are those with neurologic or physical disabilities that impair function. Neurological handicaps can be motor, sensory, emotional, or intellectual in nature. Advanced age and obesity do *not* qualify as impairments under the *Act* (Figure 2-7).

Under Title I, a dentist who employs 15 or more people for a minimum of 20 weeks annually must comply with the applicable *AwDA Title I* requirements. *Title I* specifically prohibits discrimination against a qualified individual (employment candidate) with a disability because of the disability.

What Is the Americans with Disabilities Act?

The *Americans with Disabilities Act* is a federal legal provision designed to prevent discrimination of handicapped persons. It provides a national mandate for the elimination of discrimination against individuals with disabilities and provides clear, strong, enforceable standards addressing discrimination against disabled people. The *AwDA* is broken down into five titles; *Titles I* and *III* have the greatest relevance to dental practices.

- *Title I* – eliminates discriminating employment policies.
- *Title II* – prohibits discrimination against the disabled in the use of public transportation.
- *Title III* – requires that public accommodations operated by private entities not discriminate against individuals with disabilities.
- *Title IV* – prohibits discrimination against the disabled in the area of communication, especially the hearing and speech impaired.
- *Title V* – contains miscellaneous provisions regarding the continued viability of other state or federal laws providing disabled persons with equal or greater rights than the *Act.* This section also prohibits state or local governments from discriminating against individuals with disabilities.

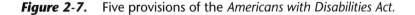

Figure 2-7. Five provisions of the *Americans with Disabilities Act.*

Title III of the *Act* covers public accommodations (any facility operated by a private entity whose operations affect commerce, including a professional office of a healthcare provider). A dental office is a public accommodation under the *Act.* A public accommodation includes a private home to the extent it is used for a professional office of a health care provider, including a dental practice.

Under *Title III,* the dental office is a public accommodation and thus may not refuse to provide access and services to any person because he or she is disabled. The obligation not to discriminate is placed on anyone who owns, leases (or leases to), or operates a place of public accommodation.

The underlying principles of the nondiscrimination requirements of *Title III* include:

- equal opportunity for the disabled to participate,
- equal opportunity for the disabled to benefit, and
- the opportunity for the disabled to receive benefits in the most integrated setting possible.

Violations of the *Act* include civil monetary penalties: up to $50,000 may be assessed for the first violation and up to $100,000 for subsequent violations. In addition, a violator (dentist) may be ordered to provide services that are found to have been wrongfully denied (Figure 2-8).

Necessary Office Renovations

The *AwDA* does *not* require the dental practice to remove all barriers to accessibility, providing a plan of priorities is established. The Department of Justice recommends barriers be removed based upon the following priorities:

- *Access to premises* – providing access from public sidewalks, parking, and public transportation. This can be done by providing wider entrances, ramps, and accessible parking spaces, including designated handicapped spaces.
- *Access to service areas* – creating physical access, as well as eliminating barriers for the visually and hearing impaired.
- *Access to restrooms* – widening doorways, installing ramps, adding appropriate signage, widening toilet stalls, and installing grab bars in restrooms.
- *Access to other areas of the practice* – providing equal services to the disabled.

Equipping the Office to Accommodate Handicapped Patients

The Department of Justice recommends the following modifications to barriers that may be readily achievable under the *Americans with Disabilities Act:*

- Installing ramps
- Installing curb cuts (areas where the sidewalk dips down to accommodate wheelchairs or vehicles)
- Designating handicapped parking spaces
- Installing raised letters and Braille on elevator controls
- Providing visual alarms
- Widening doors and doorways
- Installing grab bars
- Installing raised toilet seats and large stalls
- Repositioning paper towel dispensers in restrooms
- Installing paper cup dispensers at existing water fountains
- Eliminating high-pile, low-density carpeting

Figure 2-8. Department of Justice recommendations.

Reception areas should feature built-in counters and patient interview areas accessible to accommodate handicapped persons. Providing a clipboard or table is an acceptable alternative if counter areas cannot be reached by wheelchair patients.

For access to treatment rooms, if steps exist between treatment and service areas, ramps must be provided for wheelchair patients. Portable ramps are acceptable if permanent ramps are not readily available. A portable ramp should be equipped with handrails and a slip-proof surface.

Office restrooms should have raised letters and Braille symbols to designate men's and women's restroom doors. Widening of doors and doorways, installing grab bars, raised toilet seats, full-length mirrors, and repositioning of paper towel dispensers are required to make restrooms accessible to the handicapped. Water fountains must also be made accessible when readily achievable. If water fountains cannot be lowered, a paper cup dispenser must be installed within reach of a wheelchair-bound patient's chair.

A minimum of one wheelchair-accessible telephone must be made available when public telephones are provided inside the facility. Should the public telephone not be accessible, a private telephone should be made available. Signage must be posted near the public telephone to indicate the location of the private telephone.

Audible alarms must be installed for the visually impaired and visual alarms should be installed to alert the deaf. Directories should be posted to designate the location of visual alarms.

All attempts should be made by the dental team to integrate handicapped patients into the practice. No service can be denied, nor can an individual patient be excluded, segregated, or otherwise treated differently than other patients, simply because the patient has a handicap.

Auxiliary aids and services included in the *AwDA* include qualified interpreters, notetakers, printed instructions and materials, telephone handset amplifiers, assistive listening devices, telephones compatible with hearing aids, or other effective methods of making visually delivered materials available to hearing-impaired patients. Auxiliary aides for visually impaired patients may include taped texts, Braille materials, and large print materials. Additional fees may *not* be charged by the practice for providing any auxiliary aid or service, barrier removal, or any other measures necessary to ensure compliance with the Act.

To help offset costs of upgrading or modifying physical structures in the office, Congress instituted the *Disabled Access Credit* (form 8826) whereby 50 percent of eligible access expenditures up to $10,250 may be deducted or depreciated from taxes.

Risk Management Strategies to Prevent Malpractice

Dental legal and ethical concerns continue to grow as the number of dental **malpractice** suits rises. The dental office manager must keep in mind that while lawsuits cannot be eliminated or prevented, the risk for potential must be kept to a minimum. Thus the term **risk management** is used as a *preventive strategy* to reduce this potential. While the dentist is the primary person listed in a malpractice suit or complaint, *all members of the dental team may be held* **liable.**

The wise office manager is alert to strategies for risk management and ways to reduce the potential for malpractice suits against the practice. The following concepts are important to the office manager in preventing malpractice suits.

Negligence

In most states, a dentist is **negligent** when he or she "does an act within his or her profession that a responsible dentist would not do, or fails to do an act that a reasonable dentist would do." If a lawsuit is filed against the dentist, it must be shown that the dentist acted negligently and that this negligence was the cause of the patient's injury for an award to be made. While the dentist, as primary care practitioner and/or owner of the practice, is most often the one against whom a suit is filed, any member of the dental staff may also be held accountable for negligence or harm done to a patient.

In most states, if the dentist is found negligent, this is an adverse action, reported to the **National Practitioner Data Bank.** The adverse action is also automatically reported to the respective dentist's State Board of Dental Examiners. The National Practitioner Data Bank functions as a national reporting entity to track and monitor complaints against licensed health care professionals. The Health Care Quality Improvement Act of 1986 brought about the creation of the National Practitioner Data Bank as a central repository for information on paid malpractice claims and adverse reports of health care licensees.

Standard of Care

An unsatisfactory treatment outcome does *not* confirm negligence on the part of the dentist. It must be proved that the dentist provided treatment that deviated from an applicable **standard of care,** and that this departure resulted in the injury sustained by the patient.

In health care, there are no "absolute" standards of care; rather, treatment guidelines that a dentist with the same knowledge, skill, and care in the same community would provide. Thus, the standard of care may be interpreted to mean, "Did the dentist act reasonably at the time and under the circumstances?"

Abandonment

Abandonment of patients is considered under **unprofessional conduct** in most State Dental Practice Acts. Under this provision, the dentist may not withdraw treatment of a patient unless both reasonable notice of the withdrawal and replacement dentist(s) are offered to the patient. Failure to treat a patient whose needs are apparent and for which the opportunity to treat the patient exists may be considered negligence.

Burden of Proof

In a malpractice case, the **burden of proof** requires that the patient seeking to impose liability against the dentist must supply the more convincing evidence that the dentist's action caused resulting harm or injury.

Elements of Malpractice

All dental staff are legally obligated to adhere to the dental standards set forth in the State Dental Practice Act. As an example, many states require all dental staff to have CPR certification with periodic updates. In addition to familiarity with the terms set forth in the State Dental Practice Act, the dentist and staff must possess an awareness of treatment procedures and protocols that fall within the standard of care. Failure to perform any of the following may be considered cause for malpractice:

- the first element is a *duty to act.* A health care practitioner has a legal and ethical duty to respond when treatment is required.
- the second element is an act of *omission* or an act of *commission.* The first means failing to carry out something that should be done to prevent harm or injury; the second means committing an act that contributes to or directly causes harm or injury. Failure to provide CPR to a patient in cardiopulmonary arrest would be an act of *omission.* Separating a root canal instrument and leaving it in the tooth without informing the patient would be an act of *commission.*
- The third element is *proof of injury or harm* caused to a patient of record. This most commonly refers to physical injury, but may include emotional or psychological harm.
- The fourth element is *failure to act as a reasonable, prudent person* was the **proximate cause** of the patient's injuries. An example would be spilling acid etch material on a patient's skin resulting in burning (Figure 2-9).

Causes of Malpractice Suits

More than two-thirds of the claims made in health care malpractice suits are directly relevant to *unexpected outcomes* or *unrealistic expectations* perceived by the patient. The following sequence of events is often what leads up to a patient's filing of a malpractice suit:

1. A dental problem occurs that may be unexpected but not unusual under the circumstances.
2. The patient is unhappy with the situation or result.
3. The patient contacts the dentist for clarification or solutions.
4. The patient is dissatisfied with attempts or explanations made by the dentist about the perceived problem or result associated with treatment.
5. The patient files a malpractice suit.

Another very common reason patients file malpractice is *poor communication* on the part of the dentist or staff.

Failure to diagnose or inform the patient of a specific clinical finding is another common reason for filing a malpractice suit.

Failure to diagnose and treat or refer for treatment to a specialist is common cause for malpractice.

Failure to explain treatment options and the expected, realistic outcome and/or consequences of nontreatment is another cause of malpractice suits.

Elements of Malpractice

Four elements must be proven to establish malpractice:

1. Duty to act or render care
2. Acts of *omission* or *commission*
3. Injury to the patient
4. Failure to act was the proximate cause of the patient's injury

---

Figure 2-9.   Elements of malpractice.

Steps to Prevent Malpractice

The following risk management steps are important to reduce the possibility of a lawsuit against the dentist. The dental office manager must ensure that these steps are followed and that all team members are familiar with them.

1. Always obtain **informed consent**, written, signed, and dated, prior to proceeding with treatment. If the patient is a minor or is mentally incompetent, the office manager must obtain informed consent from a parent or guardian on behalf of the patient. (*Note:* Implied consent, which simply interpreted means the patient sits in the dental chair and implies that she or he consents to whatever dental treatment is needed, is no longer sufficient.)

   Informed consent is more than obtaining permission to examine or treat a patient. It includes the ailment, disease, or problem; the recommended treatment and the risks involved; alternative treatments and the risks; inadequate or nontreatment risks; and fees (Figure 2-10).

2. Always obtain a thorough medical and dental history, signed and updated; again, if the patient is a minor or is mentally incompetent, request this information from a parent or guardian. It is the office manager's responsibility to update this information at each recall visit, or at a minimum, annually.

3. Make sure all records are complete and accurate. These include up-to-date radiographs, a written treatment plan, diagnosis, and dated treatment progress notes. Also document that the reasons for recommended treatment were explained to the patient, including possible complications of delayed treatment or noncompliance with recommended treatment. Document that all treatment options and their corresponding **prognoses** were explained to the patient. If the patient elects *not* to accept or proceed with recommended treatment, request that she or he sign a detailed, dated waiver rejecting treatment and stating that he or she understands the consequences.

4. Document all patient complaints, comments, and reasons for seeking treatment.

5. Always enter chart notations in ink. Never erase, cover up, white out, or attempt to amend records. If an error is made, draw a single line through the error, initial and date the error, and make the correction immediately next to the original chart entry. All staff members, including the dentist, must initial chart entries.

DENTAL TREATMENT CONSENT FORM

*Please read and initial the items checked below
and read and sign the section at the bottom of form.*   Patient Name_____

☐ **1. WORK TO BE DONE**

I understand that I am having the following work done: Fillings_____ Bridges_____ Crowns_____ Extractions_____
Impacted teeth removed_____ General Anesthesia_____ Root Canals_____ Other_____
(Initials_____)

☐ **2. DRUGS AND MEDICATIONS**

I understand that antibiotics and analgesics and other medications can cause allergic reactions causing redness and swelling of tissues, pain, itching, vomiting, and/or anaphylactic shock (severe allergic reaction).   (Initials_____)

☐ **3. CHANGES IN TREATMENT PLAN**

I understand that during treatment it may be necessary to change or add procedures because of conditions found while working on the teeth that were not discovered during examination, the most common being root canal therapy following routine restorative procedures. I give my permission to the Dentist to make any/all changes and additions as necessary.   (Initials_____)

☐ **4. REMOVAL OF TEETH**

Alternatives to removal have been explained to me (root canal therapy, crowns, and periodontal surgery, etc.) and I authorize the Dentist to remove the following teeth _____ and any others necessary for reasons in paragraph #3. I understand removing teeth does not always remove all the infection, if present, and it may be necessary to have further treatment. I understand the risks involved in having teeth removed, some of which are pain, swelling, spread of infection, dry socket, loss of feeling in my teeth, lips, tongue and surrounding tissue (Paresthesia) that can last for an indefinite period of time (days or months) or fractured jaw. I understand I may need further treatment by a specialist or even hospitalization if complications arise during or following treatment, the cost of which is my responsibility.   (Initials_____)

☐ **5. CROWN, BRIDGES AND CAPS**

I understand that sometimes it is not possible to match the color of natural teeth exactly with artificial teeth. I further understand that I may be wearing temporary crowns, which may come off easily and that I must be careful to ensure that they are kept on until the permanent crowns are delivered. I realize the final opportunity to make changes in my new crown, bridge, or cap (including shape, fit, size, and color) will be before cementation.   (Initials_____)

☐ **6. DENTURES, COMPLETE OR PARTIAL**

I realize that full or partial dentures are artificial, constructed of plastic, metal, and/or porcelain. The problems of wearing these appliances have been explained to me, including looseness, soreness, and possible breakage. I realize the final opportunity to make changes in my new dentures (including shape, fit, size, placement, and color) will be the "teeth in wax" try-in visit. I understand that most dentures require relining approximately three to twelve months after initial placement. The cost for this procedure is not included in the initial denture fee.   (Initials_____)

☐ **7. ENDODONTIC TREATMENT (ROOT CANAL)**

I realize there is no guarantee that root canal treatment will save my tooth, and that complications can occur from the treatment, and that occasionally metal objects are cemented in the tooth or extend through the root, which does not necessarily affect the success of the treatment, I understand that occasionally additional surgical procedures may be necessary following root canal treatment (apicoectomy).   (Initials_____)

☐ **8. PERIODONTAL LOSS (TISSUE & BONE)**

I understand that I have a serious condition, causing gum and bone inflammation or loss and that it can lead to the loss of my teeth. Alternative treatment plans have been explained to me, including gum surgery, replacements and/or extractions. I understand that undertaking any dental procedures may have a future adverse effect on my periodontal condition.   (Initials_____)

I understand that dentistry is not an exact science and that, therefore, reputable practitioners cannot fully guarantee results. I acknowledge that no guarantee or assurance has been made by anyone regarding the dental treatment which I have requested and authorized. I have had the opportunity to read this form and ask questions. My questions have been answered to my satisfaction. I consent to the proposed treatment.

Signature of Patient_____ Date_____

Signature of Parent/Guardian if patient is a minor_____ Date_____

#21153 – Medical Arts Press 1-800-328-2179

Figure 2-10. Informed consent form. *(Reprinted courtesy of Medical Arts Press 1-800-328-2179.)*

6. If an additional treatment note is required, enter it on a new line in the chart, with *addenda* and the date.

7. Never discard inactive patient records. Store them in a separate, secured area and retain them for a minimum of 30 years.

8. Always keep treatment, financial, and personal patient documentation and records on separate forms.

9. Follow a uniform chart entry system to ensure conformity and lessen the likelihood of omission of relevant information.

10. If records are requested or subpoenaed, forward quality duplicates—never the originals!

11. Never berate another dentist's treatment. Clinical records and related discussion and documentation should include only the patient's condition as diagnosed, objective observations, patient's comments relating to the situation, and the recommended necessary treatment plan.

12. Document in the record all telephone conversations with patients, referring specialists, and authorized prescriptions.

13. Use sequentially numbered prescription pads with carbon paper or carbonless copies, and always place one copy into the patient's record.

14. Document all cancellations, late arrivals, and disappointments in the record.

15. Enter the dates of all radiographs and other diagnostic casts in the record.

16. Enter specific postoperative instructions or note that standard postoperative instructions were given to the patient.

17. Note the type (generic or brand name) of materials used for all dental procedures.

18. Never make treatment guarantees! Instead, educate patients that their active participation and cooperation have a substantial effect on the success of their treatment outcomes.

When an Accident Happens or a Patient Complains

If an accident occurs, especially resulting in undue injury or harm to a patient, or if there is a complaint by a patient, the office manager should say nothing. Instead, she or he should alert the doctor to the nature of the patient's injury or complaint and let the doctor handle it appropriately.

When a Patient Declines or Discontinues Treatment

In the event that a patient chooses to discontinue planned treatment, the doctor feels it is in the patient's best interest to seek dental treatment elsewhere, or the practice has been sold, great caution must be taken in releasing the patient from the doctor's care. This is to reduce the likelihood of the patient's claiming **abandonment** and also to ensure that the patient finds another treating dentist of record.

The practice should take the following steps in dismissing a patient:

1. Send a certified, return–receipt request letter to the patient. Include two copies and request the patient sign, date, and return one copy. This provides written documentation for the office files.

2. Include in the letter the reasons for treatment discontinuance, such as failure to comply with recommended treatment or home care, or failure to pay for services.

3. The dentist should offer to be available to provide emergency care only, for the next 30 calendar days, from the date of the certified letter.

4. The dentist should also offer to forward copies of the patient's records to the new treating dentist or to make copies available for the patient to pick up, upon receipt of a written, signed, and dated request. The office should provide legible copies and may charge a reasonable fee to provide these copies. The practice legally owns the records, although patients have access to them.

5. The dentist should also provide the names of several practitioners or clinics available to provide continued care.

Patient Confidentiality

Guarding the doctor-patient relationship is key to confidentiality. Anything that is said, done, or written in the office is considered confidential. As such, names, addresses, telephone numbers, the nature of treatment, medical or financial history, and diagnosis are not generally disclosed to the public or to other private agencies.

For insurance-processing purposes, most claim forms contain a statement and signature line requiring that the patient or responsible party agree to the release of treatment information, medical-dental history, and other pertinent information (such as Social Security Number) for the claim to be processed. When in doubt, the office manager should always check with the doctor before releasing information.

In the event that a patient requests release of treatment records or the dentist refers the patient to a specialist for further evaluation or treatment, the office should obtain a written, signed, and dated request from the patient or the new treating dentist of record. The office may release copies of the original clinical records and duplicates of dental radiographs. The office should retain the original patient records for 30 years.

Patient Confidentiality and the Fax Machine

The introduction of the fax machine has created patient-confidentiality concern among healthcare professionals. The following guidelines are helpful when considering whether to fax records for timeliness (Figure 2-11).

Reporting Suspected Domestic Abuse

All 50 states have laws requiring licensed healthcare professionals, including dentists and dental hygienists, to report cases of suspected domestic abuse, including violence **(active abuse)** and neglect **(passive abuse).**

Under these laws, the licensed dental professional is immune from prosecution for reporting abuse, even when no legal foundations confirm the suspected or alleged abuse. The dental assistant is a nonlicensed dental professional and is not bound by law to report cases of domestic abuse or neglect; however, she or he should take the dentist aside and report her or his observations and suspicions.

Domestic abuse most often involves child abuse, but also encompasses **spousal abuse** (sometimes referred to as "battered woman syndrome" or battery), committed against a marital partner or significant other living in the same household, or elder abuse against a geriatric relative or dependent.

Signs and Symptoms of Domestic Abuse

Defined as maltreatment or negligent treatment by a partner, guardian, other caretaker, or relative, abuse and neglect may result in broken bones, cigarette burns, human bite marks, starvation, or sexual molestation. Abuse is an act of *commission;* neglect is an act of *omission.*

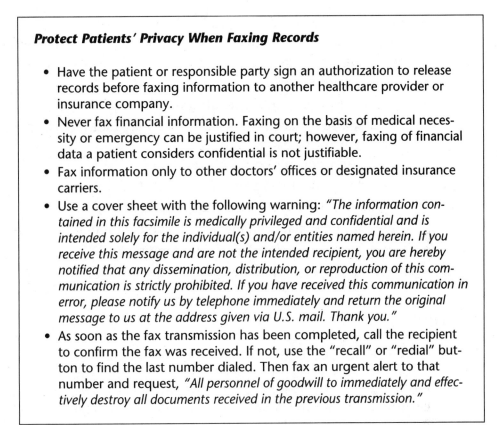

Protect Patients' Privacy When Faxing Records

- Have the patient or responsible party sign an authorization to release records before faxing information to another healthcare provider or insurance company.
- Never fax financial information. Faxing on the basis of medical necessity or emergency can be justified in court; however, faxing of financial data a patient considers confidential is not justifiable.
- Fax information only to other doctors' offices or designated insurance carriers.
- Use a cover sheet with the following warning: *"The information contained in this facsimile is medically privileged and confidential and is intended solely for the individual(s) and/or entities named herein. If you receive this message and are not the intended recipient, you are hereby notified that any dissemination, distribution, or reproduction of this communication is strictly prohibited. If you have received this communication in error, please notify us by telephone immediately and return the original message to us at the address given via U.S. mail. Thank you."*
- As soon as the fax transmission has been completed, call the recipient to confirm the fax was received. If not, use the "recall" or "redial" button to find the last number dialed. Then fax an urgent alert to that number and request, *"All personnel of goodwill to immediately and effectively destroy all documents received in the previous transmission."*

Figure 2-11.   Steps to ensure patient confidentiality when faxing records.

Child Abuse

The majority of all domestic abuse cases involve trauma to the mouth, face, or head. **Child abuse** must be at least suspected when a child appears with any of the following unexplained signs:

- battering or other injuries around the head or neck
- black eyes or blood clots in the nostrils
- bruises on edentulous ridges or severe lacerations of the oral mucosa

- oral radiographs that exhibit healed or recent fractures
- venereal warts or HIV-associated lesions, such as oral candidiasis, which indicate sexual abuse
- a fractured nose or broken or avulsed teeth
- cigarette burns, rope or electrical cord burns
- bald or sparse spots on the scalp, which may indicate hair-pulling or dragging by the hair
- bruise patterns or cuts on the face and ears
- ruptured or punctured eardrum
- unexplained broken or bruised nose or jaw
- bruises or finger marks on the neck or submandibular throat area
- scars or burns on the head, neck, lips, or tongue
- bite marks on any part of the body

Spousal Abuse

In cases of suspected domestic abuse, especially of battered women, the dentist should interview the patient privately, away from the suspected abusing partner. The dentist should attempt to help correct the problem in a professional, compassionate, and nonjudgmental manner. Continued failure to correct a problem of abuse or neglect, or an attitude of indifference about it, must raise suspicion.

Reporting and Documenting Procedures

Any licensed healthcare provider may report suspected domestic abuse or neglect by telephone, in person, or by written documentation. Failure to do so is a crime punishable by fine and imprisonment. Required information to file a report of suspected abuse should include:

- the name, address, age, gender, and approximate height and weight of the victim
- the name and address of the responsible custodial adult or partner
- a description of the physical and emotional abuse and/or neglect of the patient

- supporting clinical evidence of previous negligence or injuries
- supportive information that may help establish the cause or source of the injuries
- the nature of the patient's condition or injuries
- photographs, radiographs, or sketches showing the nature and location of the injuries

Some state protective agencies permit the healthcare provider to photograph injuries without a parent or guardian's consent (in cases of abuse of a minor). Other states allow only designated authorities to photograph injuries arising from abuse.

It is also important to carefully document in the patient's record any findings of suspected neglect or abuse, including:

- the time and date the injury was observed and noted
- the location and number of injuries
- the color and size of each lesion, bruise, or injury
- the caretaker's verbal response to the cause of the injuries

It is also essential to have another individual witness the examination and initial or co-sign the documentation to corroborate any suspected domestic abuse or neglect.

Skill-Building for Success: Student Activities

These optional activities and exercises are designed to help the student put into practice information learned in the chapter.

1. Discuss and describe the difference between ethics and jurisprudence. Give an example of each.

2. List and describe the duties of the State Board of Dental Examiners and give at least three reasons why its role is important.

3. Break into groups for 10 minutes and prepare a list of reasons dental assistants and office managers should maintain high ethical standards. Brainstorm an incident in which a dental assistant or office manager may be asked to make an ethical decision and provide possible solutions. Share your conclusions with the class.

4. Break into groups for 10 minutes and prepare a list of three scenarios of legal and/or financial aspects of hiring practices. Determine if each was legal or illegal. Share your scenarios and decision with the class.

5. Discuss the following scenario: You are hired in an office where the dentist permits staff to perform functions that are outside the scope of the State Dental Practice Act. You become aware of this. What should you do? Discuss this as a group.

6. A patient of record calls to make an appointment for a disabled family member. What information should the office manager obtain prior to making the appointment? What, if anything, should you do before scheduling the appointment? Is it illegal for the office to refuse to treat a disabled patient?

7. List 10 things the staff can do to lower the practice's potential for a malpractice suit.

8. An eight-year-old child is seated for his first appointment. He appears to have signs of neglect or abuse. What measures should the office manager or dental assistant take? Should she report her suspicions directly to the authorities? Why?

Skills Mastery Assessment: Post-Test

Directions: Select the response that best answers each of the following questions. Only one response is correct.

1. In a dental malpractice suit, which of the following people may be held liable?
   a. the dentist
   b. the dental hygienist
   c. the office manager
   d. any/all of the above

2. The dental office manager must keep in mind that while lawsuits cannot be eliminated or prevented, the potential risk must be kept to a minimum.
   a. True
   b. False

3. Dental jurisprudence:
   a. requires understanding of regulations that pertain to the State Dental Practice Act
   b. is a philosophy of law or a set of legal regulations enacted by the legislature
   c. contains rules and legally allowable duties that may be performed by qualified dental personnel
   d. all of the above

4. Ethical requirements are considered a lower standard than jurisprudence requirements.
   a. True
   b. False

5. The State Board of Dental Examiners:
   a. protects the health, safety, and welfare of the public
   b. regulates the criteria for dental licensees within the state
   c. monitors licensees and enforces discipline for noncompliance
   d. all of the above

6. Under supervision rules stipulated in the State Practice Act, the dentist:

   a. is responsible for all acts delegated to and performed by staff (within the law)
   b. must be physically present in the office when staff perform direct supervision procedures
   c. must be physically present in the office when staff perform general supervision procedures
   d. a and b only

7. The office manual:

   a. provides a single source of written office policies and procedures
   b. provides a standard of fairness for all employees
   c. is considered legally binding (an implied contract) in most states
   d. all of the above

8. Under current employment laws, the dentist as employer is required to select the most qualified candidate for the position.

   a. True
   b. False

9. All of the following fall under current law regarding employee records *except:*

   a. the records are confidential
   b. the records may not be released to the employee upon the death of the dentist or sale of the practice
   c. the records become property of the employee when she leaves the practice
   d. all of the above fall under current law

10. The Americans with Disabilities Act covers patients with:

    a. advanced age
    b. obesity
    c. any physiological disorder or condition
    d. a history of domestic abuse

11. When dismissing a patient from the practice the dentist should:
    a. be available to provide emergency dental care for the next 90 days
    b. inform the patient in person
    c. inform the patient in writing by certified mail with return receipt requested
    d. hold the clinical records until the patient's balance has been paid

12. Child abuse may be suspected when the patient appoints with which of the following?
    a. cigarette burns, rope or electrical cord burns
    b. black eyes or blood clots in the nostrils
    c. venereal warts or HIV-associated lesions, such as oral candidiasis, indicating sexual abuse
    d. any/all of the above

13. To protect a patient's privacy before faxing records, the office manager should:
    a. have the patient or responsible party sign an authorization to release records
    b. call the patient's insurance carrier for third-party verification
    c. push the redial button on the fax machine
    d. destroy the fax cover sheet

14. When filing a report of suspected domestic abuse, the dentist should include:
    a. the nature of the patient's condition or injuries
    b. the name and address of the responsible custodial adult or partner
    c. supporting clinical evidence of previous negligence or injuries
    d. all of the above information should be included

15. If an accident occurs or a complaint is made by a patient, the office manager should:
    a. say nothing
    b. alert the dentist to the nature of the patient's injury or complaint
    c. attempt to calm the patient down and offer a refund for the treatment rendered
    d. a and b only

16. The dental professional may be found negligent:
    a. when he or she commits an act a responsible dentist would not do
    b. when he or she fails to do an act that a reasonable dentist would do
    c. if the patient's injury was caused by the dentist
    d. all of the above

17. Which of the following does *not* fall within the scope and authority of the National Practitioner Data Bank?
    a. it is a national reporting entity that tracks and monitors complaints against licensed healthcare professionals
    b. it is a central repository for information on paid malpractice claims and adverse reports on healthcare licensees
    c. it has the power to revoke dental licenses
    d. all are within the NPDB's scope of authority

18. Under a provisional employment agreement the assistant may earn unemployment benefits.
    a. True
    b. False

19. If the dental office manager suspects a patient suffers from some form of domestic abuse, she or he should:
    a. take the dentist aside to discuss her or his observations and suspicions
    b. report the case to the appropriate authorities
    c. attempt to take corrective action by interviewing the patient away from the caregiver
    d. all of the above

20. As total compensation, the dental office manager's package may include:
    a. an hourly or weekly salary and paid vacation and holidays
    b. a uniform allowance
    c. reimbursement for attending continuing education courses
    d. any/all of the above

References

American Dental Association works with Dentists to Comply with Americans with Disabilities Act. [Press release]. (1992, December). Chicago: American Dental Association.

Baker, S. (1997, August). Charting for the jury. *Dental Economics*.

Curtis, E. (1997, October). Code words: A newly revised ADA manual highlights five ethical duties. *Inscriptions*.

Curtis, O. (1997, December). Salary packages. *Dental Economics*.

Detecting and reporting child abuse: Guidelines to determine symptoms of abuse and neglect. (1998). Office of Oral Health, Arizona Department of Health Services: Author.

Devore, C. (1993, October). Disabilities Act gives protection to a wide range of disabled workers. *RDH*.

Dietz, E. (1996). Gearing up to accommodate the handicapped patient: What is the Americans with Disabilities Act and how does it impact the dental team? [Home study program]. Rolling Hills, CA: Healthwatch.

Dietz, E. (1997). Career enrichment: Expand the skills you have to create the job you want. Falls Church, VA: National Association of Dental Assistants.

Dietz, E. (1997). Detecting and reporting domestic violence: Manifestations to the head and neck. (Home study programs). Fair Oaks, CA: GSC.

Guarding the files: Your role in maintaining the confidentiality of patient records. (1996, August). *Journal of the American Dental Assistants Association Vol 127*.

Protzman, S. (1996, May/June). The dental assistant's management of medical emergencies. *Journal of the American Dental Assistants Association Vol 127*.

Quinn, J. (1992, Fall). Chart your practice course with an office manual. *Preview*.

Sfikas, P. (1996, January). What dentists need to know about employment law. *Journal of the American Dental Assistants Association Vol 127*.

Rhode, J. (1992, July/August). Protect yourself! Ten gems for developing your practice "at-will" policy. (Newsletter). Phoenix, AZ: *SmartPractice*.

Tekavec, C. (1997, December). What is doctor/patient privilege? *Dental Economics*.

Torres, H., Ehrlich, A., Bird, D., and Dietz, E. (1995). *Modern Dental Assisting* (5th ed.). Philadelphia: Saunders.

Chapter 3

Hazard Communication and Regulatory Agency Mandates

- **The Role of Government Agencies and How They Affect the Dental Office**
- **Complying with Local, State, and Federal Regulations**
  Occupational Safety and Health Administration (OSHA)
  The Centers for Disease Control and Prevention (CDC)
  The Environmental Protection Agency (EPA)
  The Food and Drug Administration (FDA)
  The Organization for Safety and Asepsis Procedures (OSAP)
- **Hazard Communication Program**
  Product Warning Labels and Stickers
  Material Safety Data Sheets (MSDSs)
  Staff Training
  Training Recordkeeping
  Reducing Hazards in the Dental Office
  Handling Hazardous Materials
  Barrier Devices
- **Bloodborne Pathogens Final Standard**
  Exposure-Control Plan
  Engineering and Work Practice Controls
  Universal Precautions
  Personal Protective Equipment

Handling and Laundry of Reusable PPE
Decontamination of Surfaces
Waste Management
Hepatitis B Vaccination
Exposure Incidents
Recordkeeping
- **Waterline Biofilms**
- **Fire and Emergency Evacuation Procedures**
  Signage Requirements
- **The Safety Coordinator's Duties**

Learning Objectives

Upon completion of this chapter, the student will achieve an 80 percent or higher score on the Skills Mastery Assessment Post-Test *covering the following material.*

1. Describe the role of government regulatory agencies and how they affect the dental office.

2. Describe the importance of maintaining a hazard communication program and the necessary components.

3. List ways to reduce hazards inherent in the dental office.

4. Describe the necessary procedures for handling hazardous materials in the dental office.

5. List and describe the components of OSHA's *Occupational Exposure to Bloodborne Pathogens Final Rule* and the responsibilities of the dental team to implement them.

6. Describe the necessary recordkeeping required by the government with regard to staff training.

7. Describe the inherent dangers of biofilms in dental unit waterlines and methods to reduce the risk of cross-contamination associated with them.

8. List fire and other required emergency evacuation procedures.

9. List the duties of the office safety coordinator.

Key Terms

biofilms

biohazard warning label

Bloodborne Pathogens Final Standard

Centers for Disease Control and Prevention (CDC)

engineering controls

Environmental Protection Agency (EPA)

exposure-control plan

exposure incident

Food and Drug Administration (FDA)

Hazard Communication Standard

hazard communication program

hepatitis B vaccination

injury log

Material Safety Data Sheets (MSDSs)

medical waste

occupational exposure

Occupational Safety and Health Administration (OSHA)

Organization for Safety and Asepsis Procedures (OSAP)

personal protective equipment (PPE)

potentially infectious materials (PIMs)

universal precautions

work practice controls

The Role of Government Agencies and How They Affect the Dental Office

A variety of government agencies have responded to the demands of patients for protection from diseases and other potential hazards associated with dental care. New regulations, as well as stringent enforcement of older regulations, require dental practices to follow guidelines and recommendations set forth by government regulatory agencies.

Complying with Local, State, and Federal Regulations

There are many government regulatory agencies that affect the way dental practices protect their employees and patients from potential hazards associated with dental treatment.

Occupational Safety and Health Administration (OSHA)

The **Occupational Safety and Health Administration (OSHA)** requires employers, including those in the healthcare profession, to establish and carry out a wide range of procedures designed to protect employees, implement and maintain employee exposure-incident records for the duration of employment plus 30 years, and provide specific **personal protective equipment (PPE)** to protect staff from infectious diseases and other potential hazards.

OSHA's *Bloodborne Pathogens Final Standard* covers all dental employees who could *reasonably anticipate* coming into contact with blood, saliva, and other **potentially infectious materials (PIMs)** during the course of employment. It is designed to help them minimize occupational exposure to bloodborne illnesses and thus protect them from possible resulting illness.

The Centers for Disease Control and Prevention (CDC)

The **Centers for Disease Control and Prevention (CDC)** have set forth specific guidelines for infection control and disease containment. Although the CDC does not have enforcement power over dental practices, OSHA is charged with investigation and enforcement of the CDC's guidelines.

The Environmental Protection Agency (EPA)

The **Environmental Protection Agency (EPA)** regulates and registers certain products used in dental practices, including surface disinfectants. The EPA requires products to undergo and pass specific testing requirements prior to approval for registration.

The Food and Drug Administration (FDA)

The **Food and Drug Administration (FDA)** regulates marketing of medical devices that include equipment and disposables items. The FDA reviews product labels for false or misleading information and sufficient directions for use. As such, the FDA regulates many chemical *germicides* used as *antiseptics, disinfectants, drugs* and *sterilizers.*

The Organization for Safety and Asepsis Procedures (OSAP)

The **Organization for Safety and Asepsis Procedures (OSAP)** is a national organization of teachers, practitioners, dental healthcare workers, and manufacturers and distributors of dental equipment and products. OSAP develops and communicates standards and information on aseptic technique to dental practices and educational institutions to assist them in the efficacy of their infection control programs.

Hazard Communication Program

The focus of OSHA's **Hazard Communication Standard** is the *Employee Right to Know Law,* which addresses the right of every employee to know the possible dangers associated with hazardous chemicals and other related hazards in the workplace. This law also requires employers to provide methods for corrective action.

To comply with the Hazard Communication Standard, the dentist must develop and implement a *written* compliance program. This must include an exposure-control plan (including the *Bloodborne Pathogens Final Standard*), a written **hazard communication program,** waste and sharps handling and management, and injury and illness prevention (Figure 3-1).

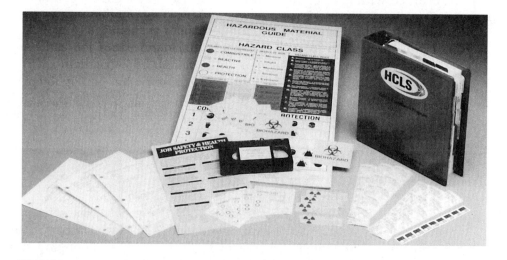

Figure 3-1. Each office must maintain an office manual with exposure-control plans, training material, hazard communication, and OSHA-required employee records. *(reprinted courtesy Medical Arts Press 1-800-328-2179)*

The dentist must also ensure that hazardous chemicals used in the office are properly labeled and hazardous substances have corresponding **Material Safety Data Sheets (MSDSs)** available for staff training and review.

The dentist must designate a program coordinator to provide staff training to new employees and once annually thereafter. The dentist must also maintain and update the written hazard communication program, develop ways to reduce hazards in the office, and provide a safe means for handling of hazardous materials.

Product Warning Labels and Stickers

Warning labels must be attached to containers, products, or other hazardous materials used in the dental office. The most common of these include *mercury* (used in silver filling material to create *amalgam*), *nitrous oxide sedation gases* (used for conscious sedation), and *chemicals for dental X-ray processing* (developer and fixer).

The label or sticker must contain appropriate warnings by hazard class, including routes of entry (into the body) and target organs (of the body) that may be affected. Product labels must contain the identity of the chemical, the appropriate hazard warnings, and the name and address of the manufacturer (Figure 3-2).

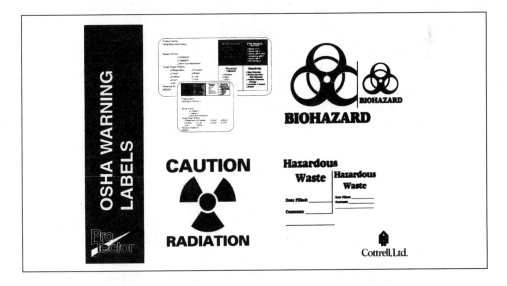

Figure 3-2. OSHA warning labels for hazardous products and devices, and biohazard labels for hazardous waste. *(reprinted courtesy Cottrell Ltd.)*

A container properly labeled when received from the manufacturer or supplier does not require an additional label. The exception for labeling is single-use or single-dispensing items or products.

All members of the dental team should familiarize themselves with the labels of hazardous substances and be aware of how to clean up spills or handle other emergencies that may arise when handling these products. The most basic elements required for a hazardous spill kit include absorbent material (to soak up the liquid), a scooping device (for a "no-touch" method to pick up the material), and a hazardous waste bag with a bio-hazard warning label. Hazardous products moved from one container to another must have an appropriate warning label or sticker affixed to the new container.

If a mercury spill occurs, the American Dental Association recommends the following procedure:

1. If the spill occurs on a carpeted floor, *do not* use a vacuum cleaner to pick up the droplets.
2. Pick up all visible droplets with a narrow bore tubing connected by a wash-bottle trap to a low-volume aspirator on the dental unit. The trap bottle connections keep the mercury in the bottle and prevent it from being sucked back into the dental unit.
3. Use adhesive tape to clean up small spills.
4. If the spilled mercury droplets cannot be reached, dust sulfur powder on them to form a film coating on the top of the droplets.
5. Keep a commercial mercury spill kit on hand. Follow the manufacturer's directions and document the circumstances of the spill with the date and cleanup procedure used (Figure 3-3).

Material Safety Data Sheets (MSDSs)

Material Safety Data Sheets (MSDSs) provide written information about the content and potential hazard of specific products. Each product that has a potential hazard must have a corresponding MSDS on file in the office. By law, MSDSs must be provided by manufacturers or suppliers of products. It is the dentist's responsibility, however, to ensure that these sheets are obtained and kept up to date (Figure 3-4).

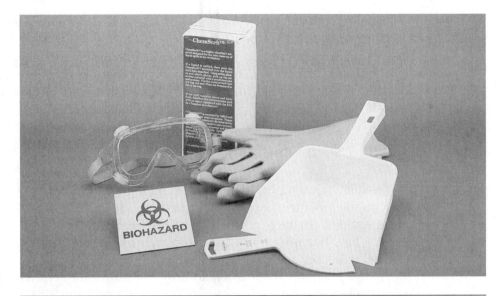

Figure 3-3. Hazardous Material spill kit. *(courtesy SmartPractice, Phoenix, AZ.)*

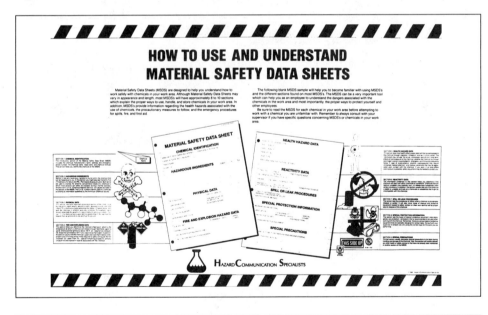

Figure 3-4. Material Safety Data Sheets (MSDSs) provide a wealth of product information. OSHA requires all dental personnel understand how to use MSDSs and where they are located in the office.

MSDSs must always be available and accessible to all employees for review. They must be kept updated.

The dental office must also maintain a *Hazardous Materials Log,* which is a list, file folder, or binder of all hazardous materials or substances used in the office, as well as the location of each item and the quantity on hand (Figure 3-5).

Staff Training

By law, the dentist must provide staff training regarding potential hazards inherent in the practice, including hazardous chemicals. This training must be provided for new employees at the beginning of employment, whenever a new hazardous material is introduced into the office, and at least annually thereafter.

The dentist is legally responsible to provide this training, however she or he may delegate training responsibilities to the office manager, safety coordinator, or other team member.

Material Safety Data Sheets

OSHA requires each MSDS contain:

- Identification (chemical and common names)
- Hazardous ingredients
- Physical and chemical characteristics (boiling point, vapor pressure, etc.)
- Fire and explosion data
- Health hazard data
- Reactivity data
- Spill and disposal procedures
- Protection information
- Handling and storage precautions, including waste disposal
- Emergency and first aid procedures
- Date of preparation of the MSDS
- Name and address of the manufacturer

Figure 3-5. OSHA required information on MSDSs.

Training must include:

- hazards of chemicals and proper handling
- the operation where hazardous chemicals are used
- the availability of MSDSs
- an explanation of the labeling of hazardous chemicals
- an explanation of OSHA regulations

OSHA also requires that hazard communication training include methods and observations that may be employed to detect the presence or release of a hazardous substance in the work area (for example, continuous radiation, nitrous oxide monitoring devices, or particular odors associated with chemicals).

Physical and health hazards of these chemicals used in the work area must be addressed (for example, avoidance of handling mercury with ungloved hands, or the potential for acid etch to burn skin or clothing).

Training must also include measures employees can take to protect themselves from hazardous materials, such as personal protective equipment (PPE) (wearing of protective gloves, eyewear, and face masks), which must be supplied by the employer, in appropriate sizes for all clinical staff members.

The employer is also responsible for explaining the details of the hazard communication program, including the labeling system, the use and nature of MSDSs, and ways employees can obtain and use the appropriate hazard information for their safety.

Employee training may be conducted at staff meetings, using audiovisuals, lectures, and video tapes, or at continuing education courses offered through accredited providers. It is essential that the training be conducted in such a way that employees understand the information presented and that their questions are answered. Training must be conducted at no cost to employees, during standard working hours.

Training Recordkeeping

Verification of training must also be documented, indicating when and where the training took place and those present. Training records should be maintained for a minimum of three years. Training records must be available to employees upon request for review and copying.

A *training summary* should contain a description of the content and nature of the training, the names of those in attendance, and the qualifications of the safety training coordinator.

In the event the practice is sold or transferred, employee records must be transferred to the new owner. If the practice is permanently closed due to death or retirement of the dentist, these records should be offered (in writing) to the National Institute for Occupational Safety and Health (NIOSH) 90 days prior to the anticipated close of the office (Figure 3-6).

Reducing Hazards in the Dental Office

It is the responsibility of all members of the dental team to reduce hazards and the potential for hazards. This can be accomplished by:

- keeping the number of hazardous materials to a minimum
- reading all product labels and following directions for use
- storing hazardous chemicals in their original containers

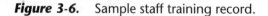

Staff Training Record

Date: _____ To: _____ From: _____ Hours: _____

Title/Topic: _____

Training Summary: _____

_____

_____

Safety Coordinator/Trainer: _____

Staff Members Present _____ Job Title_____

_____

_____

_____

Figure 3-6. Sample staff training record.

- keeping containers tightly closed or covered when not in use
- avoiding the combination of two or more known hazardous chemicals; for example, mixing household chlorine bleach with ammonia may cause an explosion; inhaling the fumes may be fatal
- wearing appropriate personal protective equipment (PPE) when using hazardous chemicals or when there is potential for accidental exposure on contact with body fluids
- washing and thoroughly drying hands before and after wearing gloves
- keeping the office well ventilated and avoiding skin contact with known hazardous substances
- keeping a functional fire extinguisher in the office
- knowing proper cleanup procedures in the event of a chemical spill
- disposing of all hazardous chemicals and other substances in accordance with MSDS instructions or the product label (Figure 3-7)

Exposure-Minimizing Form for Employees

Each dental staff member who has the potential to contact hazardous chemicals or products should have an Exposure-Minimizing Form on file. When the job duties or descriptions change, the form must be updated to reflect the changes or additions.

Name: _____ Job: _____ Date: _____

Tasks Assigned	Engineering Controls	Work Practice Controls	PPE Used

---

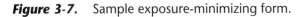

Figure 3-7. Sample exposure-minimizing form.

The *Exposure-Minimizing Form* provides a guide to outline and define the primary tasks performed by each staff member who may, as part of the nature of the job, have potential or probable exposure to hazardous substances or PIMS.

The "Tasks Assigned" column should have general tasks, such as instrument sterilization, sanitizing and setting up treatment rooms, and disinfecting and wrapping cases to send to outside dental labs.

The "Engineering Controls" column should include those types of equipment or safety devices used in the office to help minimize risks to employees. These may include scrubbing instruments with an ultrasonic cleaner, placing plastic barriers on treatment room equipment, or installing a protective shield on the model trimmer.

The "Work Practice" column should include measures taken by staff to eliminate or reduce exposure. These might include instructions such as avoid touching contaminated instruments directly, avoid inhaling glutaraldehyde fumes, or avoid using a model trimmer without a shield and face mask.

The PPE used for these procedures should be listed for each task, for example: gloves, eyewear, mask, and gowns.

Handling Hazardous Materials

Because contact with hazardous materials is inevitable when working in the dental office, there are measures the dentist and staff can take to protect themselves. The most significant measure is using personal protective equipment (PPE), part of the universal precautions mandated by OSHA.

As part of the hazard communication program the office must have a written procedure for handling and disposing of used or outdated materials that cannot be poured down the sanitary sewer or treated as routine or medical waste. These items include, but are not limited to, outdated X-ray solutions, vapor sterilization fluid, lead foil from dental X-ray packets, scrap amalgam, and glutaraldehyde solution with a concentration of higher than 2 percent.

Dental team members must be instructed on how to handle spills and cleanup of hazardous substances and chemicals. In the event of an accidental spill, staff should follow the manufacturer's instructions (found on the label or on the MSDS) and wear appropriate PPE.

Barrier Devices

To prevent the spread of infectious diseases, disposable barriers must be placed to protect splash surfaces likely to be contaminated during the course of patient treatment. Protective barriers include plastic sleeves over dental tubings, covers on dental light handles, light switches, patient chairs, and X-ray machine tubeheads (Figure 3-8) (Figure 3-10).

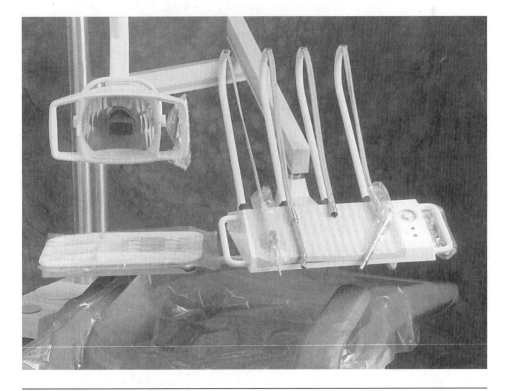

Figure 3-8. Disposable plastic barriers and sleeves protect the dental light handles, handpieces, air-water syringes, and the dental chair from cross-contamination of infectious diseases. *(reprinted courtesy Perio Support Products, East Irvine, CA.)*

Dental X-ray films are available prewrapped in clear plastic outer packets to facilitate sound infection-control practices (Figure 3-9).

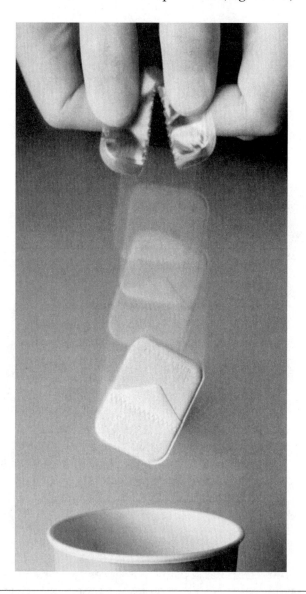

Figure 3-9.   Dental X-ray film supplied in protective barrier packet (ClinAsept™) provides sound infection control. *(reprinted courtesy Eastman-Kodak Company, Rochester, NY.)*

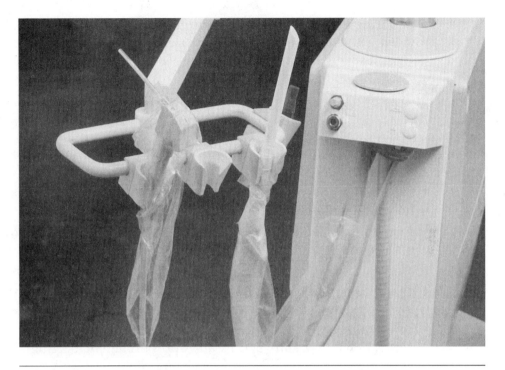

Figure 3-10. Disposable plastic tubing protects the air-water syringe and oral vacuum tubings. *(reprinted courtesy Perio Support Products, East Irvine, CA.)*

Bloodborne Pathogens Final Standard

The Bloodborne Pathogens Final Standard is the most significant OSHA regulation affecting healthcare practices. To proceed, it is first necessary to understand the term *bloodborne pathogen*; a bloodborne pathogen is any disease-producing microorganism that may infect a human. A microorganism is so small it may only be seen under a microscope.

The *Bloodborne Pathogens Final Standard* is designed to protect dental office employees by limiting occupational exposure to blood, saliva, and other PIMS (potentially infectious materials), which otherwise could result in transmission of bloodborne pathogens to healthcare workers. The standard covers all employees who could be exposed to blood or saliva during the performance of job duties. As such, employees must be informed of or provided with the following (Figure 3-11).

Exposure-Control Plan

Every dental office must have a written **exposure-control plan** designed to identify tasks, procedures, and job classifications where occupational exposure takes place. The exposure-control plan must include:

- copies of all government regulations with an understandable explanation of the contents
- a general explanation of the nature and symptoms of bloodborne diseases including but not limited to AIDS, hepatitis, and tuberculosis
- an explanation of the ways bloodborne pathogens are transmitted
- an explanation of how to recognize tasks and other activities that may involve exposure to blood, saliva, and other PIMS
- an explanation of how to use measures known to prevent or reduce occupational exposure, specifically appropriate engineering controls, work practices, and PPE
- information on the types of PPE available, including proper use, location, removal, handling, decontamination, and disposal
- an explanation of the criteria for selecting PPE
- information on hepatitis B vaccine, including its efficacy, safety, method of administration, and the benefits of vaccination; also that the vaccine will be offered at no charge to all full-time employees by the employer
- instructions on what to do if an accidental exposure incident occurs, including how to report it and the necessary medical follow-up
- information on the post-exposure evaluation and follow-up, which the employer must provide at no charge, following an exposure incident
- an understandable explanation of the signs, labels, and color coding required for PIMs and other potentially harmful substances in the dental office

The practice compliance checklist may be helpful to the practice in complying with infection control and hazard communication requirements.

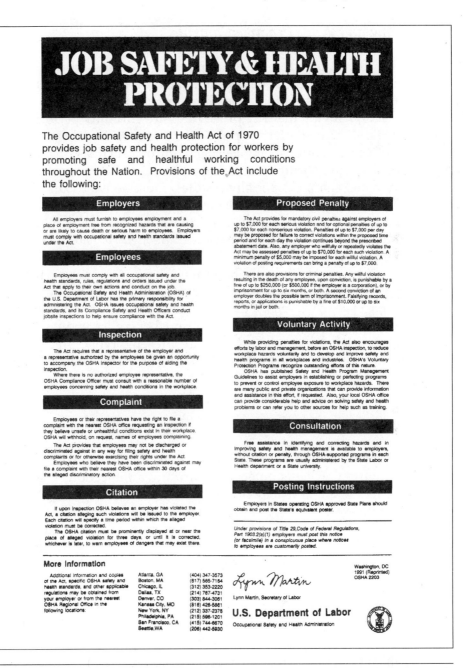

Figure 3-11. OSHA's provisions of the Occupational and Health Act of 1970 provide job safety and health protection for workers, including against bloodborne pathogens.

Engineering and Work Practice Controls

The office must use proper **engineering controls,** which means the use of specific equipment or devices that facilitate prevention of accidental exposure, such as recapping needles, for example. **Work practice controls** means changing the way procedures are currently performed to ensure a higher degree of safety or protection from accidental exposure.

OSHA requires engineering controls such as making appropriate handwashing facilities available and accessible to all staff members. Contaminated sharps, especially needles, must be handled appropriately and disposed of to prevent accidental exposure. A minimum of *one eyewash station* must be immediately available to all personnel. Other engineering controls applicable to dentistry include *high-volume evacuation* and use of *dental dam.*

OSHA guidelines also require work practice controls that prohibit eating, drinking, smoking, applying cosmetics or lip balm, and handling of contact lenses in areas of the office where there is a reasonable potential for occupational exposure. All food and beverages should be stored separately from areas where PIMS are present. Work practice controls also include proper handwashing, handling of sharps, and containment of regulated waste.

Universal Precautions

Following **universal precautions** means treating each and every patient as though she or he is potentially carrying an infectious disease. Therefore, the same standards of personal protection must be observed when treating *all* patients.

Universal precautions emphasize employing engineering and work-practice controls to reduce the level of contamination that may be involved during an accidental exposure.

Personal Protective Equipment

Personal protective equipment (PPE) consists of a minimum of four items, which must be worn by chairside personnel, who have a reasonable potential to come into contact with infectious diseases. These items are gloves, protective eyewear, face masks, and gowns. In some instances a faceshield may be substituted for protective eyewear, but does not replace a face-mask. If preferred, goggles may be used as protective eyewear over contacts or prescription eyeglasses. If eyeglasses are worn as PPE, they must have sideshields to protect the wearer from splatter or contact with infectious microorganisms (Figure 3-12).

Lab coat, gowns, or other PPE may be disposable or made of cotton-polyester. If, during the course of a procedure, a disposable item is torn or

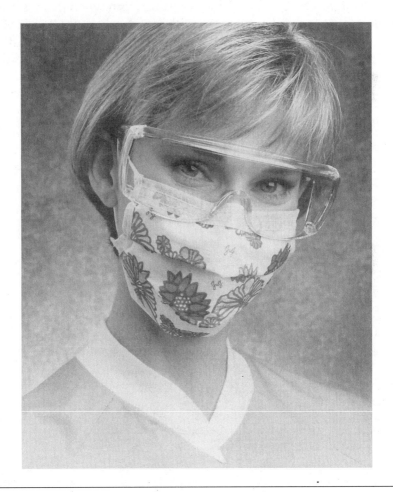

Figure 3-12.   Clinical personnel must wear personal protective equipment for performing chairside and other clinically related tasks. *(reprinted courtesy Johnson & Johnson Medical, a Division of Ethicon, Inc.)*

saturated, the procedure must be stopped and the torn or visibly saturated item must be replaced.

When working away from chairside, such as in the dental lab or when preparing instruments for sterilization, all personnel must protect themselves by wearing PPE. In this instance, however, the gloves must be made of heavy nitrile material (as opposed to single-use exam gloves worn when treating patients) that may be sterilized and reused.

The employer must provide, maintain, and ensure use and laundry of PPE, at no charge to staff. PPE must be worn when there is a potential for an employee to come into contact with blood, saliva, or other PIMs (Figure 3-13).

In instances where dental staff have known sensitivities to PPE—for example, allergy to latex gloves—the employer must provide alternatives, such as vinyl gloves or cotton glove liners.

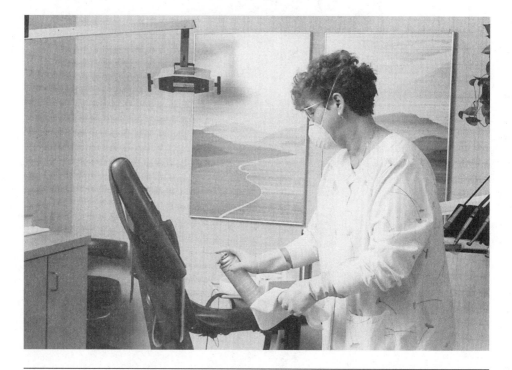

Figure 3-13. The dental assistant disinfects the treatment room. Note the personal protective equipment: utility gloves, mask, eyewear, and outer protective clothing.

Handling and Laundry of Reusable PPE

Handling of reusable PPE (that which is not single-use disposable) must be kept to a minimum. It is the dentist's responsibility to provide laundry or dry cleaning services for reusable lab jackets, lab coats, or scrubs worn during invasive procedures. Contaminated laundry in the office must be placed into containers that are red or labeled with the biohazard symbol.

Dental staff may not wear outer protective clothing worn for invasive procedures to and from the office; nor may they wear it when leaving the office during the day, such as during a lunch hour.

Furthermore, outer protective clothing may be laundered following the manufacturer's directions and with standard laundry detergents. It may not, however, be done with other household clothing. They must be laundered at the office or at a commercial laundry. Staff may launder their clothing worn underneath outer protective clothing at home.

Decontamination of Surfaces

The standard requires the office to have a written cleaning and maintenance schedule for surfaces and other areas that may become contaminated with blood or saliva. This description should outline how equipment and treatment rooms are decontaminated.

Reusable containers that become contaminated must be cleaned and disinfected when visibly soiled. Likewise, plastic covers and barriers must be replaced when contaminated (between patients). Equipment being shipped for repair, such as dental handpieces, must be decontaminated or labeled as a biohazard.

Waste Management

Regulated **medical waste** is defined as liquid or semi-liquid body fluid. This includes any items in the dental office contaminated with regulated waste (for example, cotton rolls or gauze) that release *bioburden* (contaminated hazardous or infectious material) when compressed, items caked with dried body fluid that have the potential to release bioburden during handling, contaminated sharps, and pathological and microbial wastes containing body fluid.

Any type of disposable sharps, that is, any item capable of puncturing the skin (needles, scalpels, burs, orthodontic wires), must be disposed of in puncture-resistant, color-coded or labeled, red, closable, leakproof containers. Sharps disposal containers must be located as close as possible to where sharps are used in the office. They must also be kept upright and must be closed during transport.

Needles must not be recapped by hand; nor may they be broken or sheared by hand prior to disposal. Instead, dental personnel should use either a one-handed "scoop" technique or a mechanical device designed to hold the needle sheath. For procedures involving multiple injections using a single needle, the unsheathed needle should be placed in a location where it will not become contaminated or contribute to unintentional percutaneous (through the skin) needlesticks between injections (Figure 3-14).

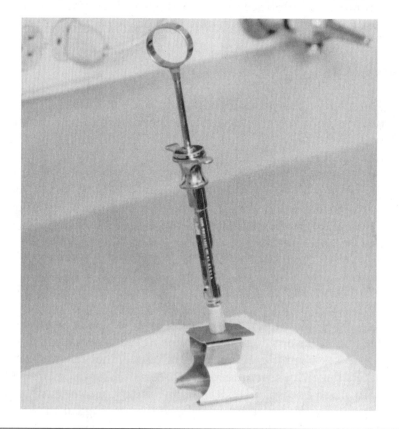

Figure 3-14.   Needles must be recapped using a one-handed scooping method or a mechanical device.

OSHA requires that full sharps containers be removed from the office within seven days of reaching the "fill line" on the container.

Other regulated waste products, including those items saturated or visibly caked with blood or saliva, must be disposed of in closable, leak-proof bags or covered containers. The containers must either be red or have a **biohazard warning label** or tag affixed to them, readable from a distance of five feet (Figure 3-15).

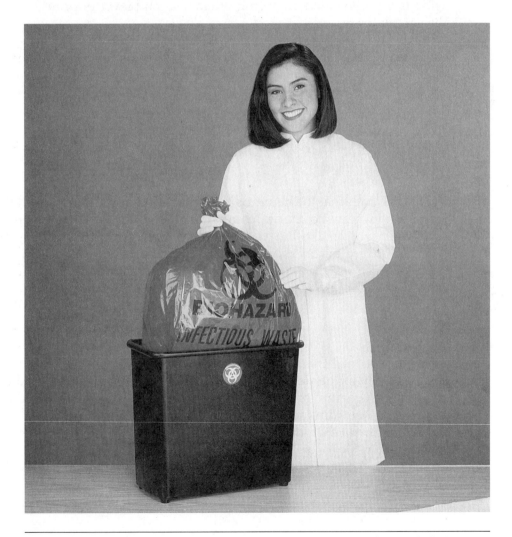

Figure 3-15. Medical waste must be labeled and properly disposed of. *(courtesy SmartPractice, Phoenix, AZ.)*

Contaminated refuse must be kept covered at all times. Receptacles must have a properly fitting lid, preferably one that can be opened using a foot pedal.

Waste receptacles should be kept closed to prevent air movement and the spread of contaminants. They should be lined with sturdy plastic bags that can be removed without touching the interior of the liner. Dental personnel must wear PPE when changing waste receptacle bags. Double-bagging is recommended because it offers a second layer of protection if the bag breaks or tears.

Laws vary by state and region regarding proper waste transport and tracking. The office manager should check with the local regulatory agency in her area for additional regulations. As a general requirement, medical waste must be disposed of within 30 days in offices that generate less than 20 pounds of medical waste per month.

Hepatitis B Vaccination

OSHA requires that the **hepatitis B vaccination** be administered to all full-time employees who are at potential risk for bloodborne pathogens. The employer must make the vaccination available to all employees at no charge. In rare instances where employees refuse the vaccination, they should sign a waiver acknowledging their refusal of the vaccine and that they do not hold the employer liable for the consequences.

Exposure Incidents

If a member of the dental team sustains an **exposure incident,** directly related to the nature of employment, the dentist is required to follow specific steps. According to OSHA, an exposure incident consists of "specific eye, mouth or other mucous membranes, non-intact skin or parenteral contact with blood or other PIMS that directly results from the performance of an employee's duties." Most common examples of **occupational exposures** occur when dental staff accidentally cut themselves on a contaminated dental instrument or sustain a needlestick injury from a contaminated anesthesia syringe.

If an exposure incident occurs, the staff member should stop immediately and report the incident to the office manager and to the dentist. If the exposure involves the hands, the employee should remove the gloves. The injury should be treated with scrupulous first-aid measures, including the following.

If the affected area is bleeding, the staff member should squeeze it gently until a small amount of blood is released. Next, the person should wash her or his hands thoroughly with antimicrobial soap and water that is comfortably warm to hot. After drying the hands, she or he should apply a small amount of antiseptic to the area and cover it with a bandage.

The employer must follow specific OSHA guidelines, including providing an independent medical evaluation of the exposure incident. The employer must:

- document the route or routes of exposure and how the incident occurred
- attempt to identify the source individual (the patient who was treated using the specific instruments or needle) if possible
- obtain the results of that patient's blood tests, if available
- with informed consent of the affected employee, have the employee's blood collected and tested. *Note:* By law, the dentist-employer is *not* entitled to know the results of the employee's blood test, only whether the employee is fit to return to work
- obtain medically necessary injections, such as gamma globulin, hepatitis B vaccine booster, and/or possibly a tetanus booster
- see that appropriate post-exposure counseling is provided for the employee
- ensure that any additional follow-up as recommended by the attending physician is completed

An employee who sustains an exposure incident may choose to decline the exposure incident follow-up, but must sign a disclaimer waiving the employer's responsibility for future results or side effects. This documentation must be recorded on an *OSHA 200* log form in offices having more than 10 employees. In those with fewer than 10 employees, the event must be documented (Figure 3-16).

Exposure Incident Report Form

Employee: _____

Date: _____

Place and Time of Incident: _____

Those Present: _____

Route of Exposure: _____

Description of the Exposure Incident: _____

_____

_____

Engineering Controls in Place: _____

_____

Work Practice Controls Employed: _____

_____

List PPE used at time of Exposure Incident: _____

_____

Source Patient: _____

Was Source Patient Tested?   ☐ Yes   ☐ No

HIV Status: ☐ Positive   ☐ Negative

Name of Lab: _____

Date of Testing: _____

Employee Tested?   ☐ Yes   ☐ No

If Employee Refused, was Waiver signed: ☐ Yes   ☐ No

Explain: _____

Post-Exposure Prophylaxis: _____

Physician's Follow-Up: _____

Physician's Written Opinion on File?   ☐ Yes   ☐ No

Figure 3-16.   Sample exposure Incident report form.

Recordkeeping

Medical records of staff must be kept confidential and must be retained by the dentist for the duration of employment plus 30 years. They should include the names and social security numbers of all employees, copies of all employees' hepatitis B vaccination records, and any other medical records pertinent to the employees' ability to receive the vaccination, circumstances surrounding any exposure incidents, and documentation of all follow-up procedures, including the treating physician's written opinion.

Waterline Biofilms

Biofilms can be found virtually anywhere moisture and a suitable solid surface exist. They are composed of millions of microorganisms that accumulate on surfaces inside moist environments. These film-forming microbes excrete a glue-like substance that anchors them to metals, plastic, tissue, and soil particles. Biofilms attach themselves to the inner surfaces of plastic tubings used to keep handpieces cool and supply air-water syringes, where they create an ideal environment for growth.

This results in a nearly stagnant condition of the tubing's inner wall surface, even when water actively flows through the tubing. A vast number of bacteria, fungi, and viruses living inside dental units become highly concentrated, significantly increasing a patient's susceptibility to transmissible diseases.

To avoid the build-up of dental unit waterline biofilms, the CDC, the ADA, and OSAP recommend dental personnel flush their dental unit waterlines at the start of each day and between patients.

To help reduce bacterial counts, the ADA suggests dental professionals follow these guidelines to improve the quality of water in their lines and minimize disease transmission:

- at the start of each day, run and discharge water from the dental unit waterlines for several minutes
- run highspeed handpieces to release air and water for 20–30 seconds after each patient

- always follow the manufacturer's instructions for proper maintenance of handpieces and waterlines
- consider other options to improve water quality such as special filters, chemical therapeutics, and separate water reservoirs

Fire and Emergency Evacuation Procedures

OSHA requires the employer to have a written fire safety policy, consisting of training in the use and maintenance of fire extinguishers (Figure 3-17). A diagram must be provided that clearly marks the exit routes in the event of a fire. Posting of emergency telephone numbers for police, fire, and rescue is also required.

Written evacuation and safety procedures should be provided in areas susceptible to severe weather conditions, including hurricanes, tornadoes, floods, and earthquakes.

Signage Requirements

In addition to signage required by the Americans with Disabilities Act (refer to *Chapter 2, Legal and Ethical Issues and Responsibilities* for further information), signs should be posted to include office exits and potential exposure hazards, such as X-ray machines, ultrasonic machines, and microwaves. Exit signs must be illuminated and be a minimum of five inches. Doors to other rooms should also be appropriately marked with such signs as *"storage," "private," "not an exit,"* etc.

The Safety Coordinator's Duties

The office manager may be delegated the responsibilities of office safety coordinator or any portion of those outlined here, as part of the existing scope of duties. In this role the office manager may be responsible for any or all of the following to ensure compliance with government regulations:

- constantly review infection control, hazardous materials, and other office safety procedures and protocols

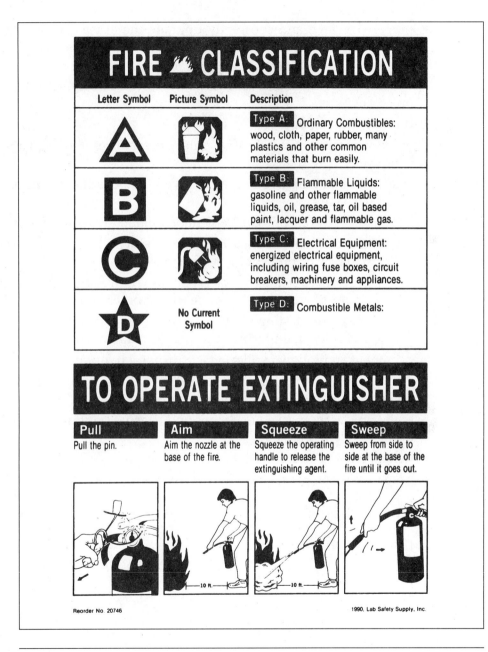

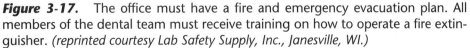

Figure 3-17. The office must have a fire and emergency evacuation plan. All members of the dental team must receive training on how to operate a fire extinguisher. *(reprinted courtesy Lab Safety Supply, Inc., Janesville, WI.)*

- prepare, review, and constantly upgrade the office exposure control plan and all manuals, including MSDSs, hazardous materials log, employee exposures, etc.
- develop procedures that provide written, step-by-step instructions for office safety
- provide training updates regularly
- monitor compliance with office safety procedures and regulations in compliance with the government
- ensure that all employees have received the hepatitis B vaccine at no charge to them
- initiate procedures for management of accidental exposure of staff
- review the circumstances surrounding accidental exposure and steps taken to reduce or prevent their recurrence
- maintain required items to protect staff as required by the government (for example, gloves, masks, eyewear) and other necessary equipment
- ensure that spore-testing of office sterilizers is done routinely and that proper biological monitoring of records is maintained
- document and follow medical waste disposal requirements
- ensure that warning labels and MSDSs, and the hazardous materials log, are maintained and updated as necessary
- maintain clearly marked exit signs and evacuation routes in the event of fire or other emergency
- maintain X-ray equipment certification
- prepare and maintain all necessary records and forms (Figure 3-18)

Practice Compliance Checklist

This checklist may be helpful to the office manager in organizing the practice's compliance list:

☐ Appropriate licenses, registrations, certificates, and OSHA posters posted in plain view of all employees

☐ X-ray certification of dental assistants posted (if required in the specific state of employment)

☐ A record of hepatitis B vaccination and any other appropriate vaccines administered

☐ Infection-control manual, hazard communication manuals, hazardous materials log, and MSDSs accessible and available for review

☐ Appropriate handwashing procedures

☐ Appropriate use of PPE, available in sizes to fit respective clinical staff members

☐ Appropriate use of barrier wraps and disposable coverings for treatment room and laboratory area

☐ Appropriate use, management, and disposal of single-use items

☐ Appropriate surface disinfection of all splash areas

☐ Appropriate aseptic technique followed by all office personnel

☐ Appropriate sterilization/disinfection of contaminated, reusable instruments

☐ Appropriate biological monitoring as recommended in the state of employment

☐ Appropriate instrument sterilization/instrument recycling area

☐ Nitrile gloves for presoaking, cleaning, and processing of instruments prior to sterilization

☐ Appropriate disposal and tracking of regulated waste and PIMs, including sharps

☐ Eyewash stations in each operatory

☐ Appropriate infection-control precautions for radiographic procedures

☐ Appropriate cross-contamination prevention in the dental laboratory area

☐ Appropriate safety checks and inspections for fire extinguishers, smoke detectors, radiation, and nitrous oxide monitors

Figure 3-18. Checklist for OSHA compliance.

Skill-Building for Success: Student Activities

These optional activities and exercises are designed to help the student put into practice information learned in the chapter.

1. List reasons why the federal government requires the dentist to maintain a hazard communication program and the necessary components.
2. List five ways to reduce hazards inherent in the dental office.
3. Describe the necessary procedures for handling hazardous materials in the dental office.
4. Develop a chart listing the necessary recordkeeping required by the government for staff training.
5. Pretend you have been assigned the role of office safety coordinator. Develop a list of duties you might be expected to perform.
6. Break into small groups. Pretend the chairside dental assistant in the office where you are employed sustained a needlestick exposure incident. She or he comes to you with a droplet of blood oozing out of her or his glove. Discuss as a group the steps you must take. Complete the sample *Exposure Incident Report Form* (see page 101). Share your steps and the contents of the form with the class.

Sample Exposure Incident Report Form

Employee: _____

Date: _____

Place and Time of Incident: _____

Those Present: _____

Route of Exposure: _____

Description of the Exposure Incident: _____

_____

_____

Engineering Controls in Place: _____

_____

Work Practice Controls Employed: _____

_____

List PPE Used at Time of Exposure Incident: _____

_____

Source Patient: _____

Was Source Patient Tested?   ☐ Yes   ☐ No

HIV Status: ☐ Positive   ☐ Negative

Name of Lab: _____

Date of Testing: _____

Employee Tested?   ☐ Yes   ☐ No

If Employee Refused, was Waiver signed: ☐ Yes   ☐ No

Explain: _____

Post-Exposure Prophylaxis: _____

Physician's Follow-Up: _____

Physician's Written Opinion on File?   ☐ Yes   ☐ No

Skills Mastery Assessment: Post-Test

Directions: Select the response that best answers each of the following questions. Only one response is correct.

1. OSHA requires employers, including those in the health care profession to:
   a. establish and carry out procedures to protect employees
   b. implement and maintain employee exposure-incident records for the duration of employment plus 30 years
   c. provide personal protective equipment (PPE) to protect staff from infectious diseases and other potential hazards
   d. all of the above

2. Hazard communication training must be provided for:
   a. new employees at the beginning of employment
   b. any time a new hazardous material is introduced into the office
   c. at least annually
   d. all of the above

3. OSHA's *Bloodborne Pathogens Final Standard* covers all dental employees who could reasonably anticipate coming into contact with blood, saliva, and other potentially infectious materials during the course of employment.
   a. True
   b. False

4. OSHA's *Bloodborne Pathogens Final Standard* is designed to help dental office employees minimize occupational exposure to bloodborne illnesses and thus protect them from possible resulting illness.
   a. True
   b. False

5. The Environmental Protection Agency:
   a. regulates and registers certain products used in dental practices
   b. requires products to undergo and pass specific testing requirements prior to approval for registration
   c. reviews product labels for false or misleading information and sufficient directions for use
   d. all of the above

6. Warning labels or stickers must contain appropriate warnings according to:
   a. hazard class, including routes of entry and target organs that may be affected
   b. the identity of the chemical and the appropriate hazard warnings
   c. the name and address of the manufacturer
   d. all of the above

7. Hazardous products moved from one container to another do not need to have a warning label or sticker affixed to them.
   a. True
   b. False

8. Which element is *not* a requirement of a basic hazardous spill kit?
   a. absorbent material
   b. a scooping device
   c. an EPA registration label
   d. a hazardous waste bag with a biohazard warning label

9. The office must maintain Material Safety Data Sheets on every product that has a potential hazard. MSDSs must:
   a. provide written information about the content and potential hazard of a specific product
   b. be provided by the manufacturer or supplier
   c. always be available and accessible to all employees for review and be kept updated
   d. all of the above

10. The *Hazardous Materials Log* must list all hazardous materials or substances used in the office, as well as where each item is located in the office and the quantity on hand.
    a. True
    b. False

11. Whether conducted by the dentist, the office safety coordinator, or the office manager, staff training must include:
    a. hazards of chemicals and their proper handling
    b. the availability of MSDSs
    c. an explanation of the labeling of hazardous chemicals and an explanation of OSHA regulations
    d. all of the above

12. Members of the dental team may reduce hazards and their potential by:
    a. reading all product labels and following directions for use
    b. avoiding the combination of two or more known hazardous chemicals
    c. wearing appropriate personal protective equipment (PPE) when using hazardous chemicals or when there is potential for accidental exposure on contact with body fluids
    d. all of the above

13. Which is *not* a requirement of the hazard communication program?
    a. having a written procedure for handling and disposing of used or outdated materials that cannot be poured down the sanitary sewer or treated as routine or medical waste
    b. instructing dental team members on how to handle spills and clean-up of hazardous substances and chemicals
    c. joining OSAP
    d. maintaining a hazardous materials log

14. To prevent the spread of infectious diseases, disposable barriers must be placed to protect splash surfaces likely to be contaminated during the course of patient treatment. Protective barriers include:
    a. plastic sleeves over dental tubings
    b. covers on dental light handles, light switches, and patient chairs
    c. dental X-ray tubeheads and outer film packets
    d. all of the above

15. Following universal precautions means:
    a. treating each and every patient as though potentially carrying an infectious disease
    b. using the same standards of personal protection when treating all patients
    c. employing engineering and work-practice controls to reduce the level of contamination that may be involved during an accidental exposure
    d. a and b only

16. Personal protective equipment (PPE) must be worn by chairside personnel who have a reasonable potential to come into contact with infectious diseases. Required PPE items include:
    a. gloves
    b. protective eyewear
    c. face masks
    d. all of the above

17. Dental sharps must be disposed of in containers that are:
    a. puncture-resistant
    b. color-coded or labeled
    c. closable and leakproof
    d. all of the above are requirements of sharps disposal

18. Sharps disposal containers must:
    a. be located as close as possible to where sharps are used in the office
    b. be kept upright and must be closed during transport
    c. not be filled above the "fill" line
    d. all of the above are requirements of sharps disposal

19. Dental personnel should use either a one-handed "scoop" technique or a mechanical device designed to hold the needle sheath for recapping.
    a. True
    b. False

20. Hepatitis B vaccination must be:

a. provided by the employer to all full-time employees who may be exposed during the course of their jobs

b. provided at no cost to employees

c. documented in the employee medical history records

d. all of the above

References

1910.132 OSHA general requirements [CD-ROM]. (1995, June 28). Washington, DC: Occupational Safety and Health Administration.

29 CFR part 1910.1030, Occupational exposure to bloodborne pathogens; Final rule. (1991, December 6). *Federal Register.*

Bednarsh, H., & Eklund, K. (1997, March/April). Universal precautions reconsidered. *The Dental Assistant, Journal of the American Dental Assistants Association.*

Controlling occupational exposure to bloodborne pathogens in dentistry. (OSHA Document 3129). (1992). Washington, DC: U.S. Department of Labor.

Dietz, E. (1998). *Career enrichment: Expand the skills you have to create the job you want.* Falls Church, VA: National Association of Dental Assistants.

Dietz, E. (1990). *Infection control: Stay on the safe side.* Phoenix, AZ: SmartPractice.

Enforcement procedures for the occupational exposure to bloodborne pathogens standard, 29 CFR 1910.1030. (OSHA Instruction CPL2-2,44C). (1992, March 6).

Gooch, B. (1996, January/February). Risk and prevention of occupational exposures to blood in dentistry. *The Dental Assistant, Journal of the American Dental Assistants Association.*

Infection control in dentistry guidelines. (1997, September). Organization for Safety and Asepsis Procedures (OSAP).

Infection control in modern dental practice (Publication #N-419). (1992). Rochester, NY: Eastman-Kodak Dental Products.

Infectious disease control in the dental office. (1997, January). Phoenix, AZ: Arizona State Board of Dental Examiners.

Kauffman, M. & Cushyner, K. (1997, March/April). Recommendations for routine immunizations of oral health care providers. *The Dental Assistant, Journal of the American Dental Assistants Association.*

Kimberly-Clark *Guide to the OSHA final rule for occupational exposure to bloodborne pathogens for dental professionals* (Publication #KL–]1441). (1993). Neenah, WI: Kimberly-Clark Corporation Professional Health Care.

Miller, C. (1998, February). Review of bloodborne pathogens standard clarifies OSHA's expectations of dental offices. RDH.

Miller, C. (1997, June). Safety coordinator's duties go beyond casual organization of safety plans. RDH.

Office safety & asepsis procedures research foundation infection control in dentistry guidelines. (1995, June). Annapolis, MD: Office Safety & Asepsis Procedures.

OSHA compliance checklist. (1997, Fall). *Preview.*

OSHA training requirements for dental and other healthcare workers. (1997, March) Annapolis, MD: OSAP Monthly Focus.

Pollack-Simon, R. (1998, February 27). *Staying current and in compliance with OSHA and infection control.* Seminar sponsored by the Arizona State Dental Association.

Wolfe, F. The low-down on PPE: What every hygienist needs to know about personal protective equipment. *RDH.*

Wyche, C. (1996, May/June). Infection control protocols for exposing and processing radiographs. *Journal of Dental Hygiene, Vol 70, 3.*

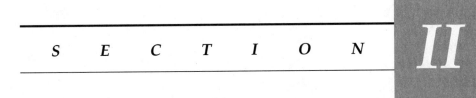

S E C T I O N   II

Practice
Communications

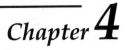

Chapter *4*

The Dental Office Manager as Patient Relations Specialist

- **Welcoming Patients as Guests**
    Prior to the New Patient's First Appointment
    Greeting the Patient
- **Reception Area Amenities**
    Creating a Comfortable Atmosphere
    Organizers and Signs
    Reading Materials
    Lighting, Ventilation, and Aroma Therapy
    Special Touches for Children
    Refreshments
    Sound System and Courtesy Telephone
- **Assisting the Patient with Necessary Forms**
    Patients' Rights
- **Introducing the New Patient to Other Team Members**
    Office Tour
- **Patient Relations: Fighting Fear with Communication**
    The Anxious Patient
    The Phobic Dental Patient
    The Angry or Agitated Patient
- **Nonverbal Communication**
    Grooming
    Posture
    Attire
    Team Portraits
- **Courtesy Communicates Respect**
    Attitude
    Etiquette

Common Courtesy and Etiquette
Follow-up Telephone Calls After Treatment
• **Offering Extended Services**

Learning Objectives

Upon completion of this chapter, the student will achieve an 80 percent or higher score on the Skills Mastery Assessment Post-Test *covering the following material.*

1. List the three goals of a patient relations policy with regard to greeting patients.
2. Describe at least seven components of a modern dental office reception area's amenities.
3. Describe the role of the office manager in assisting new patients to complete necessary forms.
4. Describe the importance of understanding and communicating patients' rights.
5. Discuss five steps to diffuse a patient's anger.
6. Discuss the differences between the anxious patient and the phobic patient.
7. Describe the protocol involved in introducing the patient to the other members of the dental team.
8. List and describe aspects of nonverbal communication and how they instill positive patient relations and perceptions.
9. Be familiar with rules of common courtesy and office etiquette.
10. Describe two important factors in making follow-up calls to patients.
11. Describe the role of the office manager in providing referrals and extended services.

Key Terms

amenities	phobia
anxiety	protocol
patient flow	

Welcoming Patients as Guests

While every member of the dental team is a patient relations representative, the office manager is most often the first and last contact most patients have with the office. It is the role of the office manager as patient relations manager to acknowledge and greet patients when they enter. Every office should have a patient relations policy for greeting and handling patients throughout the duration of their dental visits. The goals of a patient relations policy are to:

- focus on the patient rather than the procedure and on the patient's chief concerns
- manage **patient flow** (the smooth execution of the processes that take place between the time the patient arrives and is dismissed); and
- control the environment as much as possible to facilitate optimum dental care.

Prior to the New Patient's First Appointment

The expression, "You never get a second chance to make a first impression," is very appropriate in dentistry as a service profession. Prior to the new patient's first appointment, many offices have a policy of sending a variety of get-acquainted materials to facilitate the first visit and to make the new patient feel welcome. These materials include a new patient packet, a map or printed instructions about office location and parking, a copy of the practice's newsletter, office policies, and information about the doctor's professional training and background. (For further information, see *Chapter 6: Printed Communications*.)

Greeting the Patient

A patient visiting the first time may feel anxious about the choice of a new dentist, finding the building and a place to park, locating the office if it is part of a larger complex, and interacting with people whom he or she has never met.

The office manager can alleviate much of a patient's anxiety by acknowledging him or her by name within the first 30 seconds of entry into the reception area. If the patient is visiting for the first appointment, the office manager or receptionist should anticipate the new patient and introduce herself or himself by saying, *"Good morning. You must be Mr. Wilson. My name is Mary/John. We're delighted to welcome you to our practice."*

If the office is in a large complex of professional offices, she or he may further inquire, "Did you have any problems finding the office?" This helps ease any awkwardness or shyness a new patient might feel in an unfamiliar environment. It establishes the office manager as the appropriate professional to whom the patient can address questions or concerns. It "breaks the ice" by 1) beginning the conversation, 2) supplying a name for convenience in asking questions or requesting assistance, and 3) initiating the new patient's orientation, or, for a patient of record, guiding the patient to the next step of the visit.

Patients of record must also be greeted as welcomed guests. Again, immediate acknowledgment (within 30 seconds of arrival) is necessary to reassure the patient, re-establish the relationship, and keep scheduled procedures flowing on time.

An effective office manager notes on an attachment to the patient record events in patients' lives that should be recalled at the next visit, such as a vacation or a wedding in the family.

The wise office manager reviews the schedule frequently to learn the names of all the appointed patients. She or he reviews the chart to be certain appropriate follow-up comments have been noted and also indicates phonetic pronunciation, if necessary.

Greeting **protocol** can be mastered by keeping aware of the time and the schedule, monitoring the guests in the reception area closely, and rehearsing names when necessary so that they can be pronounced easily and naturally as patients enter the office.

Reception Area Amenities

The reception area is a reflection of the practice's philosophy and personality. It also assures the new patient of the doctor's values, such as treating the whole family and welcoming friends as prospective new patients. The appearance and comforting **amenities** of the reception area make a lasting impression upon patients and communicate that the dentist and staff find their comfort important.

Creating a Comfortable Atmosphere

By furnishing the reception area with hospitality in mind, the office manager can impact a patient's sense of relaxation and add an element of enjoyment to the time spent waiting for family members or awaiting her or his treatment. Many practices today have removed the frosted privacy glass of the reception window and opened the area to make a receiving counter where patients feel comfortable approaching personnel.

The traditional hard-backed chairs have been replaced by living room-like furnishings that make patients and their families feel at home.

Organizers and Signs

A coat rack, boot tray, umbrella stand, and mirror help patients feel that the office has anticipated their needs. These conveniences seem minor, but they may help put patients at ease. Signs that direct patients to information are also helpful, e.g., *"Restroom," "Receptionist,"* and *"Exit."*

Reading Materials

The reception area is the ideal place to provide educational and recreational reading materials. Most dental offices provide racks and specialized brochures that focus on a variety of oral health topics. Many also provide a video cassette player with videos featuring dental health subjects.

The creative office manager experiments with reading materials to find an appealing mix of literature. Attractively bound "coffee table" books on dental procedures or related educational topics can be displayed if space permits. Popular magazines, cookbooks, or books of cosmetic dental procedures ("before and after" makeovers of actual patients) are also popular. Reading materials must be kept up-to-date and in good shape.

Lighting, Ventilation, and Aroma Therapy

Optimal lighting should be provided in the reading areas throughout the reception area. An excellent way to determine sufficient lighting is for the office manager to seat herself or himself in the reception area from time to time with a book or magazine to see whether glare or inadequate light creates a problem.

Proper ventilation helps reduce the "dental office odors" associated with traditional practices. Many offices have automatic aroma therapy dispensing systems that release small doses of odor-neutralizing vapor into the air. Light floral and cinnamon fragrances are popular.

Special Touches for Children

Even if the practice does not serve children, some patients need to bring their children when they come for care. One of the most important comforts the office can offer for all patients is a reception area or a corner of the general reception area designated specifically for children. Adults vary widely in their enjoyment of children. A "children's corner" serves adults as well as children. Adults who would rather not deal with youngsters appreciate the separation and those who enjoy associating with children are pleasantly surprised to see that children's needs are appropriately met by the practice.

Materials that lend themselves to quiet activities for children include individual coloring sheets, crayons, and washable colored markers. Jigsaw puzzles keep many youngsters happily occupied. Toys separated into storage bins and activity boxes labeled for age appropriateness are also a welcome amenity.

Practices that treat a large number of children often have a separate reception area reserved exclusively for kids that may offer more lively diversions such as video games or popular movies on video cassette players.

As in all decisions regarding the practice, the philosophy and "image" should prevail. As practice relations specialist, the office manager is attuned to the task of supporting and promoting the practice philosophy in all the details of its management.

Refreshments

It has become increasingly common for dental practices to provide light refreshments in their reception areas as a sign of hospitality. Complimentary coffee, tea, juices, hot chocolate, and bottled water promote relaxation and make the wait seem shorter.

Sound System and Courtesy Telephone

A quality sound system is another effective way to provide a comforting, pleasant atmosphere that helps relax patients.

Just as pleasurable aromas mask smells that evoke anxiety, relaxing music can also cover sounds that might trigger fear or subconscious anxiety. Another bonus associated with background music is added privacy. Patients may feel more comfortable discussing financial arrangements or treatment options with the office manager when they sense that the music in the reception area helps make these conversations inaudible to the other patients.

Many practices also provide a separate telephone (within local calling range) as a courtesy for patients.

Assisting the Patient with Necessary Forms

The best way to ensure that all the office documentation is correct and complete is to oversee it carefully. It is the role of the office manager to offer assistance to patients when completing forms. More importantly, this assistance offers a valuable opportunity to establish a personal, caring relationship with each patient and reinforces this communication of concern at every visit.

Patients' Rights

As in any other service organization, customers (in a dental office patients are the customers or clients) have specific rights regarding information about their diagnosis and treatment. The following has been adapted from the medical/hospital system to assure patients' rights. Some practices develop their own version and display a framed copy in their reception or business office areas for patients to see, while others include it in new patient introductory forms (Table 4-1).

Introducing the New Patient to Other Team Members

When the patient has satisfactorily completed the necessary forms, the patient proceeds to the next area. The patient must be escorted to the next

Table 4-1. A Dental Patient's Rights.

Patients enrolled in our practice are entitled to be treated fairly and with dignity. We hold our patients in high regard and strive to treat them with the finest quality of care and service. Our patients are guaranteed to:

1. Be treated with respect and consideration for their dental needs.
2. Be informed of all aspects regarding dental treatment, including type of treatment and the necessity for referral, when indicated.
3. Be informed of appointment times and fee schedules.
4. A review of all financial and clinical records for himself or herself and family.
5. Obtain a thorough evaluation of oral needs.
6. Be treated as a partner in his or her care and decision making related to treatment planning and delivery and to be given an estimate of fees prior to rendering service.
7. Receive information and feel assured of quality treatment and materials.
8. Expect confidentiality of all records pertaining to dental care.
9. Receive information of the dentist's participation in various third-party payment plans.
10. Obtain appropriate referrals for consultation, specialty care, and/or second opinions.
11. Receive instruction in maintaining good oral home care.
12. Receive treatment to prevent, reduce, or eliminate future dental or related oral disease.
13. Expect continuity of treatment and to be informed of the necessity of change in treatment plan, should the need arise.
14. Be charged a fair and equitable fee for services.
15. Have appointment times maintained and respected.
16. Be treated by all members of the dental team with courtesy and respect.

room and introduced to the staff member who will be responsible for the next step in the patient's visit. The new staff member's name must be pronounced clearly, even if an earlier introduction has been made, so the patient can comfortably ask questions or initiate a conversation about the proposed treatment.

Many dental offices consider staff nametags an essential part of the team uniform and require all employees to wear them.

Office Tour

Some practices make it a matter of policy to give each new patient a tour of the office, introducing them to all team members during the tour. The benefits to the patient include increased familiarity, a sense of being treated as a partner in the health care decision-making process, increased understanding of the routine procedures of the office, and an opportunity to ask questions about sterilization procedures.

Office managers who conduct introductory tours find that patients enjoy learning more about the staff members, infection-control methods, radiography and other methods of imaging, as well as other state-of-the-art equipment used for dental care. Touring the inner workings of areas they seldom see gives patients a sense of feeling welcomed as a friend in addition to the expected professional relationship and treatment outcome.

Patients concerned about highly publicized instances of alleged disease transmission via dental equipment can see first-hand and ask questions about the practice's compliance with government-mandated guidelines for infection-control management.

Patients who suffer from irrational fear of dental care find that walking through the office helps demystify the experience and reassures them when they see other patients who are comfortable and that the staff is friendly and professional.

Parents of young children especially appreciate the tour, because it provides their family members an interesting and positive introduction to dental care. Children may be invited to take a ride in the dental chair as a preliminary introduction to the treatment room prior to their first visit.

An important part of an introductory tour is a gift for each child and a professional hand-out or information packet for the patient or prospective patient.

Patient Relations: Fighting Fear with Communication

The key to understanding patient relations is managing anxiety. Often dental patients may feel anxious about anticipated pain, temporary loss of autonomy (making one's own choices), financial concerns, and the amount of time required to maintain their oral health or treat dental disease. The office manager and members of the dental team can help alleviate these concerns through patient education and effective communication. By fostering ongoing professional relationships with patients of record as well as prospective patients, the office manager can successfully anticipate problems that prevent patients from seeking dental care. At the same time, she or he can generate referrals of new patients from satisfied patients of the practice.

The Anxious Patient

Many patients experience some degree of **anxiety** (a normal but enhanced feeling of concern) about dental appointments. The wise office manager displays awareness and a willingness to accommodate patients to help alleviate their anxiety.

The office manager can emphasize that anxiety is normal and expected, and the practice considers it a valid element of patient care to resolve patients' concerns.

There is a difference however between the anxious patient and the true dental phobic patient.

The Phobic Dental Patient

Phobia (irrational fear) refers to anxiety that interferes with normal pursuits. A true *dental phobic* is so traumatized by the environment of a dental office that it is clinically impossible to treat him or her until the phobia is controlled.

Some dentists premedicate phobic patients. Others prefer the use of *behavior modification* techniques, such as visualization, hypnosis, or biofeedback. Often the dentist contacts the patient's therapist prior to the first visit to discuss various methods of handling appointments with the phobic patient. Some phobic patients may bring along the therapist for the first visit or the first several visits, as required.

Some practices offer scheduling considerations for extremely anxious or phobic patients, such as times when there are no other patients in the office or short visits that permit the patient to adapt gradually to the fearful situation.

Other phobics are encouraged to bring a friend, spouse, counselor, or other support person. Some bring along an item that can be clutched for comfort, often a pillow, stuffed animal for a child, or a purse or briefcase for an adult. This permits the patient to bring a part of his or her comfortable environment into a frightening one and helps the phobic patient maintain a sense of control.

Some practices schedule a reception room visit (only) for the phobic patient during normal office hours. At this time, the doctor or hygienist may come out and greet the patient, but there is no treatment scheduled and the patient goes no further than the reception area.

At the next scheduled visit, the phobic patient enters the treatment room but does not sit in the chair. At a subsequent visit, the patient enters the treatment room and sits in the chair, but does not recline. Eventually, the patient will enter the treatment room, sit and recline in the chair for 10 minutes, and practice deep breathing exercises.

At the next visit the patient may undergo a preliminary oral examination. By using small, successive steps, many phobic patients gain a sense of self-mastery over anxious situations such as dental visits. In extreme cases of dental phobia, the dentist may admit the patient to the hospital where treatment is performed under general anesthesia.

The Angry or Agitated Patient

On a rare occasion, a patient may feel angry or briefly agitated about a specific event in the practice. Most often the office manager as patient relations specialist is the person responsible for addressing the patient's anger or agitation. Following are strategies the office manager can use to respectfully help diffuse the situation and calm the patient down (Table 4-2).

Nonverbal Communication

Much of the professionalism and trustworthiness the office manager aspires to express to each patient is portrayed non-verbally. The appearance (grooming, posture, and attire) of the team, the attitude and etiquette of each staff member, and the appearance of the office instill confidence and promote relaxation in patients.

Grooming

The office manager must project herself or himself as an authoritative but approachable person. Proper grooming emphasizes the professional roles of the staff members. Hair must be styled so it never needs to be touched

Table 4-2. Five Steps to Diffuse a Patient's Anger.

1. **Let the patient release the anger** – Allow him or her to vent these feelings without being interrupted. (Attempts to initially intervene or conciliate tend to fuel further anger.)

2. **Don't try to lead or second-guess where the patient is going with the conversation—instead, listen!** (Trying to anticipate his or her comments can further frustrate the patient. What most patients really want is to feel understood and to be taken seriously.)

3. **Respond only after the patient has fully vented his or her feelings** – Speak in a low, calm voice, breathing slowly to reduce your rate of speech. This reduces the tendency toward defensiveness. Use neutral comments that communicate to the patient that you care about resolving the situation. For example, *"How can I help?"* or *"This is certainly upsetting to you and I'd like to help."*

4. **Use the three Fs:** *feel, felt,* and *found* – A way to remember this is: "I know how you *feel.* I've *felt* that way myself sometimes and I've *found* this may help."

5. **Avoid the urge to argue or ventilate** – Agree with the patient that his or her feelings may be justified and then clarify the facts substantiating the patient's anger.

or attended to during the course of the professional day. Long hair must be pulled back away from the face and collar.

Because hair spray, colognes, after shave, or cosmetics trigger allergic reactions in some patients, these items must be used sparingly. During working hours the office manager must project a conservative, polished, professional image.

Particular attention must be directed to hands and nails, which must be cared for and scrupulously clean. Nails should never call attention to themselves. Nail tips should be no longer than two to three millimeters. Artificial nails (for women) are discouraged as they harbor microscopic pathogens, create undue noise on the computer keyboard, and cause fungal infections in susceptible individuals.

A reliable antiperspirant or deodorant is a must, and all practices follow the professional courtesy of informing each other privately when any area of the grooming code is breached. The professional office manager needs to be prepared to take this responsibility if she or he notices another staff member requires encouragement.

Posture

One of the most powerful nonverbal communicators is posture. By standing poised to respond and looking a patient in the eye, an office manager can immediately take control of a conversation and identify herself or himself as the person in authority. Many office managers make it a practice to kneel down to the physical level of patients in wheelchairs by pulling their chairs together to speak companionably. Similarly, sensitive office managers drop to one knee to speak to a young child, rather than towering above him or her from an intimidating height. These are examples of postures and body language that facilitate professional communication.

Slouching communicates weariness, boredom, or unwillingness to participate. Energetic, alert posture communicates helpfulness and interest. "Closed" postures, such as folding one's arms, hand-clasping or wringing, hugging oneself or crossing ankles or knees, are usually perceived as compensatory or adaptive postures. They show insecurity, hostility, or withdrawal. The practiced office manager conducts herself or himself gracefully and with authority by keeping hands open and relaxed, poised for helpful gestures or necessary actions, keeping both legs straight with weight distributed evenly. The office manager sits naturally, with both feet on the floor and ankles uncrossed.

Attire

Expectations of attire for dental office managers have undergone trend swings as with all fashions, but the standard should always reflect the role and purpose of the profession, combined with the individual practice image.

The current trend for office managers is toward the image of a financial services professional, such as a banker or broker and away from that of a clinical professional. Therefore, if all members of the dental team wear matching scrubs, as is the practice in some offices, they must be neatly pressed with creases in the pant legs. Shoes should reflect a healthcare setting rather than an athletic event.

If the office manager is permitted to make the decision, she or he should choose a formal business suit rather than scrubs as professional attire.

Team Portraits

In addition to formal introductions, many office managers hang framed portraits of the staff members, including the doctor, in the reception area. These serve as patient relations mechanisms in several ways. A picture is the obvious way to become more familiar with the dental team member. The reception area "gallery" serves as an organizational chart, showing patients at a glance the staff members' roles, their names, titles, and credentials.

Second, portraits convey a strong sense of importance to the dental team. They indicate that each member is a professional. Portraits with plaques showing the credentials of the personnel assure patients that they are in capable and trained hands.

Third, the titled portraits help patients familiarize names and associate them with faces. This makes further communication much more effective.

Fourth, portraits show team pride. Patients immediately feel a sense of community and a sense of belonging when they enter a practice with team portraits in the reception area. The portraits should be taken in "uniform" to enhance this impact.

Courtesy Communicates Respect

Courtesy and other forms of verbal communication convey a wealth of respect to patients and dental team members. This includes a positive, confident attitude, as well as etiquette and courtesy.

Attitude

No discussion on communication is complete without exploring the impact of attitude. Attitude shows in posture, grooming, attire, and spoken communication as well as unspoken messages. It is crucial to the success of the practice.

Attitudinal qualities of which a dental office manager should be self-aware include self-confidence, the quality of being genuine, a willingness to remain open to new or unfamiliar experiences, an intrinsic appreciation for the varying backgrounds or cultures of others, assertiveness, and integrity.

Etiquette

Professional etiquette falls under nonverbal communication, although much of proper etiquette involves knowing the right thing to say, the right manner in which to phrase it, and the circumstances that require specific comments. Underlying these conventions are cooperation and consideration for the common benefit of all.

First, *"please"* and *"thank you"* are always required. The office manager says, *"Follow me, please,"* when directing patients. This is more appropriate than *"Would you like to follow me?"* Each time the patient complies with a request, the office manager says *"Thank you."*

It is, however, appropriate to ask a caller if he or she would like to hold. *"Hang on,"* is never used in a dental office. The appropriate phrase is *"Would you like to hold, please?"* or *"Can you please hold?"*

Professional office managers remember patients' names. When first introduced, the name is always repeated as part of the greeting. It is repeated again when the conversation ends or the patient is released. Terms of endearment are *never* substituted for names. It is never appropriate to call a patient *"honey,"* for example. It is wise to ask the patient what variation of his or her name is preferred. Many people have strong preferences for their given names over the common nickname, while others never use their given names. It is an important aspect of etiquette to honor the patient's preference consistently.

Patients who use wheelchairs or have some other form of physical handicap should be addressed personally. It is not appropriate to speak to the escort as if the immobile person were not capable of conducting a conversation independently.

Common Courtesy and Etiquette

Simple common courtesy is required as a normal and expected part of office etiquette. While every office is slightly different in its demeanor, the following are commonsense rules of etiquette when addressing patients or team members (Table 4-3).

Follow-up Telephone Calls After Treatment

In many practices, the office manager or treatment coordinator contacts all operative and surgical patients as a courtesy to ensure there are no

Table 4-3   Commonsense Etiquette and Good Manners.

- Always use correct grammar; avoid use of slang or extensive dental jargon when speaking to patients.
- Do not interrupt another person who is speaking.
- Never eat, drink, smoke, or chew gum in front of patients.
- Avoid creating unnecessarily loud noises, such as banging of a patient history clipboard on a countertop or slamming the telephone receiver or file drawer.
- Always hand a piece of paper or chart to another person; do not toss or fling it onto a countertop or desk for the other person to pick up.
- Never lick your fingers when handling paperwork or turning pages of a document. (Think how the next person handling the papers feels!)
- Always introduce unacquainted people. Repeat each person's name for emphasis.
- If two people are engaged in conversation, avoid standing or sitting within voice range. If you must speak to one of them, leave a short note or speak to the person later.
- Always find a way to compliment or praise another person.
- Respect other people's privacy.
- If the phone rings while you are in conversation with another person, excuse yourself to answer it.
- Avoid extensive or excessive conversations that do not involve the practice or immediate patients.
- Avoid forming office cliques or engaging in subgrouping (gossiping).
- Refrain from nervous mannerisms that may distract others, such as fingernail drumming, humming, whistling, lip smacking or excessive hand or foot movement.
- Always look the other person directly in the eye when engaging in conversation.
- Recognize that people are from different cultures, walks of life, and experiences, and thus have different values.

complications and to answer questions regarding treatment. In addition to providing a reflection of care and concern for the patient, this may prevent unnecessary emergency calls or reduce risk associated with unusual bleeding or swelling, dry socket, lost temporaries, failure to regain sensation, ensuring appropriate pain control or avoiding unnecessary drug reactions. In the long run this prevents misunderstanding and hard feelings and communicates a commitment to continuity of care to all patients.

Offering Extended Services

Many practices offer extended services as an expression of hospitality that demonstrates care and concern for their patients' total well-being. Extended services may include referrals to other dental and medical members of the community for tobacco cessation counseling, weight management, massage therapy, nutrition counseling, and hypertension management. Offices may also offer or sponsor CPR classes, oral cancer screening, and chewing tobacco and sports-related injury awareness and education.

The office manager plays a vital role in providing referral information to patients under the direction of the dentist.

Skill-Building for Success: Student Activities

These optional activities and exercises are designed to help the student put into practice information learned in the chapter.

1. Think of at least three experiences you have had recently as a guest. These can represent homes of friends or strangers, businesses, or professional offices. Divide a sheet of notebook paper into two columns by drawing a vertical line down the center. Label the left column, "Negative." Label the right column "Positive." List pleasant feelings or events under the second column head, and frustrating, frightening, or awkward feelings or events under the first. Using this table as your inspiration, create a list of ideas for a comforting, pleasant, welcoming dental reception area. Use your imagination! Take turns sharing your list with the class and describe how those experiences felt.

2. Have volunteers from the class provide demonstrations of common courtesy, first using the "wrong" way, then correcting the same situation to the "right" way. Provide feedback.

3. Imagine you have been put in charge of designing a dental office of the future where patients are to be treated like important clients or guests. Make a list of amenities and other personal touches you would provide. Share your list with the class.

Skills Mastery Assessment: Post-Test

Directions: Select the response that *best* answers each of the following questions. Only one response is correct.

1. The goals of an office patient relations policy are to:
   a. focus on the patient rather than the procedure
   b. manage patient flow
   c. control the environment as much as possible to facilitate optimum dental care
   d. all of the above

2. Get-acquainted-to-the-practice materials may include any/all of the following *except:*
   a. a map or printed instructions about office location and parking
   b. office policies and information about the doctor's professional training
   c. the patient's initial diagnosis
   d. a copy of the practice's newsletter

3. All patients should be greeted as welcomed guests within _____ seconds of their arrival.
   a. 10
   b. 30
   c. 45
   d. 60

4. Special touches for the children's area of the reception room may include all of the following *except:*
   a. coloring sheets and markers
   b. jigsaw puzzles
   c. coffee table books
   d. video games

5. Proper ventilation and automatic aroma therapy help reduce the "dental office odor" associated with traditional practices.
   a. True
   b. False

6. The benefits of taking the new patient on an office tour include:

    a. an increased familiarity
    b. a sense of partnership in health care decisions
    c. an opportunity to ask questions about sterilization procedures
    d. all of the above

7. Dental anxiety is normal, while dental phobia is irrational.

    a. True
    b. False

8. Which of the following common fears is *not* typically a problem in dental practices?

    a. fear of getting lost or not being able to find the office
    b. fear of heights
    c. dental phobia
    d. fear that treatment will be too expensive

9. What is communicated nonverbally by slouching?

    a. helpfulness
    b. boredom
    c. alertness
    d. assertiveness

10. Greeting protocol can be mastered by:

    a. keeping aware of the time and the schedule
    b. monitoring the guests in the reception area closely
    c. rehearsing names when necessary so they can be pronounced easily and naturally as patients enter the office
    d. all of the above

11. Why should the office manager wear a business suit if she or he is not required to wear scrubs?

    a. she or he may be sued for impersonating a surgeon
    b. she or he should wear only flattering colors
    c. she or he is more effective at communicating if her or his attire suggests a financial services professional
    d. scrubs are too warm for most dental offices

12. Which of the following is *not* a desirable attitude for a dental office manager to cultivate?

    a. self-confidence
    b. self-absorption
    c. appreciation for diverse backgrounds and cultures
    d. assertiveness

13. Team portraits displayed in the office:

    a. help patients familiarize themselves with names and faces
    b. display team pride
    c. introduce team members as professionals
    d. all of the above

14. Most patients prefer to be addressed as "honey" or another similar term of endearment.

    a. True
    b. False

15. If two people are engaged in conversation, common courtesy dictates the office manager should:

    a. avoid standing or sitting within voice range
    b. leave a short note or speak to the person later
    c. a and b only
    d. all of the above

16. Providing follow-up care phone calls:

    a. answers patients' questions regarding treatment
    b. provides a reflection of care and concern for the patient
    c. ensures there are no postoperative complications or drug reactions
    d. all of the above

References

Dietz, E. R. (1997). Career enrichment: Expand the skills you have to create the job you want. Falls Church, VA: National Association of Dental Assistants.

Dietz, E. R. (1998, May). How to handle an angry patient. *The Explorer Vol 24, 5.* Falls Church, VA: National Association of Dental Assistants.

Finkbeiner, B., & Johnson, C. (1995). *Mosby's comprehensive dental assisting: A clinical approach.* St. Louis: Mosby.

Koren, T. (1997, September/October). The three ways to use patient education literature. *Today's Chiropractic.*

Schmidt, G., & Green, K. (1991). Market your dental practice 365 ways a year. Phoenix, AZ: SmartPractice.

Chapter 5

Marketing the Practice

Learning Objectives

Upon completion of this chapter, the student will achieve an 80 percent or higher score on the Skills Mastery Assessment Post-Test *covering the following material.*

1. Describe the need for marketing in dentistry.
2. Define and differentiate between marketing and advertising as they relate to dentistry.
3. Describe the necessity of a marketing budget and related terminology.
4. Describe the types of internal and external marketing programs as they relate to dentistry.
5. Discuss the importance and rationale of tracking results of marketing efforts in the dental practice.
6. Explain the rationale and importance of referral source management.

Key Terms

advertising	marketing
direct marketing campaign	media
event marketing	patient attributes
external marketing	patient profile(s)
focus group	target audience
internal marketing	target mailing(s)

The Necessity for Practice Marketing

During the past decade, the need for dental practices to market themselves has come about because of increasing competition for patients. Significant changes in dental practices have evolved due to a declining birth rate, reduced dental insurance benefits, an increase in managed care programs, and rising dental school enrollments. Done ethically and professionally, marketing concepts that have evolved from other professions can be used successfully to gain new patients, create an increased demand for dental services from the existing patient base, and generate additional referrals.

Advertising and Marketing Differ

Although many people use the terms interchangeably, **advertising** and **marketing** are different. Advertising is the promotion of products or services provided by a business or organization through a variety of **media**, including telephone directories, newspapers, magazines, radio, television broadcasts, and billboards.

By contrast, marketing is creating the demand, need for, or awareness of a product or service the consumer (in this case the patient) may have been unaware that he or she desired or may have been unaware was available. Today, many private fee-for-service practices effectively and ethically promote their individualized services using a variety of internal and external marketing strategies.

The American Dental Association (ADA) offers a variety of publications, reports, and booklets on ethical marketing for dental practices. Practices having questions about ethical marketing may contact the ADA for further information at (800) 621-8099.

Key Elements of Dental Marketing

Four key elements of a successful dental marketing campaign the office manager should be familiar with include:

1. create a need
2. demonstrate expertise
3. emphasize affordability
4. offer convenience

Create a Need

Only about one-half of the American population visits the dentist regularly, and fewer than that take advantage of specialized dental services. Many expanded dental services involve not only the dental treatment itself, but offer a cosmetic benefit as well. Thus, a practice that wishes to increase crown and bridge procedures, the number of units of veneers, cosmetic bonding cases, or tooth-bleaching procedures, may promote *cosmetic dentistry* as a benefit or feature associated with services available.

The patient's psychological association with elevated self-esteem, increased self-confidence, a youthful appearance, or preservation of his or her natural smile, are benefits often used to create a need for services in the mind of the patient. Terms such as "whiter teeth," "straighter teeth," "fresher breath," and "a more attractive smile," are often used as benefits of cosmetic dental procedures.

Demonstrate Expertise

After the need has been created, the marketing-minded practice must demonstrate its expertise in solving patients' perceived problems to produce desired results. Many practices stress the dentist's special education and continuing education training to meet the identified need. Patients as consumers often perceive that special training offers a higher level of service or esthetic result.

Emphasize Affordability

Practices who promote themselves through marketing programs must also provide ways to make it easy for the patient to afford their services. Types of payment plans to meet patients' needs are addressed in *Chapter 12, Managing Accounts Receivable.*

Offer Convenience

Patients as consumers expect convenience as a primary factor in making purchasing decisions. Dental practices that offer expanded treatment days, extended hours, or multiple locations, emphasize these conveniences to patients and prospective patients in their marketing campaigns. Offering a designated telephone line for new patient inquiries, an 800 number, or rapid new appointment scheduling, also emphasizes convenience.

Goal Setting

To formulate a marketing plan, the dentist and staff must first brainstorm to establish measurable goals to achieve as a result. Many practices begin by reviewing production figures from the previous year or years and then strategize to set new goals to surpass those figures.

To be measurable, a goal must be defined. An example of a definable goal is: *The practice currently schedules 30 new patients per month. Our goal for this year is to schedule 35 new patients per month. Another measurable goal might be to increase the number of units of crown and bridge per month from 45 to 50.*

If a new service is being introduced by the practice, tooth bleaching, for example, the goal might be *to make tooth-bleaching service availability known to all patients who are suitable candidates for the procedure and to enroll 30 patients to undergo tooth bleaching during the next three months* (Figure 5-1). Tracking of results appears later in the chapter.

Patient Selection

Once definitive goals have been determined, the practice then develops a **direct marketing campaign** to patients about the benefits of services, new procedures available, or to let them know that the office appreciates referral of new patients.

Monthly Goal Sheet

_____   _____

Month   Year

SERVICES:	GOAL:
Adult Prophies	_____
Amalgam Surfaces	_____
Composite Bonding Surfaces	_____
Crown and Bridge Units	_____
Endodontic Canals	_____
Quadrants of Perio Scaling	_____
Veneers	_____
Tooth Whitening Arches	_____

Figure 5-1. The practice's monthly goal sheet provides a clear and measurable understanding of the marketing direction for the practice.

The office manager selects from the computer data base a list of patients who may be candidates for a specific procedure, or who have friends, coworkers, or family members looking for a new dentist. These patients are referred to as the **target audience.**

The target audience is selected by choosing specific **patient attributes,** such as age, socio-economic status, hobbies, profession, history with the practice, ability to tolerate an elective procedure, and oral health suitable to undergo the service. Working with the dentist, the office manager determines these specific attributes and prints out a list of suitable candidates to whom to market.

The Marketing Budget

A marketing budget must be established prior to devising a marketing plan. On average, most dental offices spend 5 percent of their total overhead (expenses) on their marketing programs. If, for example, the practice has a yearly *gross* (total amount of dentistry produced and collected) of $600,000 and the *overhead* (expenses required to run the practice) is 65 percent, or $390,000, five percent of the overhead equals $19,500, as the total yearly marketing budget for the practice.

Internal Marketing

Internal marketing includes any promotional effort(s) directed toward patients and their families currently enrolled in the practice. An internal marketing campaign may encompass one or more types of promotions.

Use of the Computer in Marketing the Practice

For many office managers, the practice's computer is an invaluable tool for implementing, driving, analyzing, and tracking internal marketing programs directed toward patients. The office manager uses the practice's computer to create **patient profiles** containing specific attributes or items of information about each patient.

These patient attributes may be used for specific **target mailings** identified by patient profiles. The office manager uses the computer to print out lists of specific patients targeted to receive mailings on a topic or dental technique of interest in any category of the computer software's selection criteria.

The office manager also uses the computer to print out mailing address labels or to address postcards or envelopes directly to patients who comprise the target audience.

Event Marketing

Event marketing is a form of internal marketing that acknowledges specific events or occasions according to information contained in the individual patient's attribute profile. The office manager uses this information to acknowledge the patient's special event or reason for celebration. Examples of event marketing include patients' birthdays and anniversaries with the practice, graduations, job promotions, and retirement.

The practice may use other types of event marketing to promote itself with celebrations such as an annual office open house or to celebrate a specific number of years in practice. If an office undergoes a transition, such as a purchase or sale or entering into a partnership, this may also be announced and celebrated through an event-marketing program.

Some practices use these occasions to make special promotions or offers either to existing patients or others in the community who may be interested in becoming patients. Examples of special promotions include dollars/percent off coupons or rewards for referring new patients.

Patient Satisfaction

Some practices use patient satisfaction surveys as part of their internal marketing program to improve their existing levels of service or to create new services or improvements. The office manager uses patient satisfaction survey results to monitor, assess, analyze, and improve upon the levels of expectation and perceived quality of care reported by patients.

Patient satisfaction is measured using a variety or combination of survey tools including telephone surveys, face-to-face surveys, and mail-in surveys. (For an example of a patient satisfaction survey, see *Chapter 6, Printed Communications*.)

Focus Groups

Another method some practices use to improve levels of patient satisfaction is periodic **focus groups**. A focus group is a small group or representative cross section of the patient base.

The function of a focus group is to obtain valid feedback and suggestions from a cross-sectional representation of patients. The office manager uses this opportunity to record patients' perceptions and impressions of the practice, and to obtain specific suggestions for improvement in services or office amenities. On the dentist's direction, the office manager selects and schedules focus groups that meet as often as monthly or as occasionally as one or two times annually.

In larger practices, the focus group may be administered by an outside marketing organization in which an independent moderator asks patients specific questions about the practice and solicits suggestions for improvement.

External Marketing

External marketing is another form of practice marketing. As the name implies, it is the opposite of internal marketing and encompasses specific targeted promotions to people outside the practice or prospective patients, i.e., those people who may, as a result of receiving marketing messages targeted directly to them, inquire about becoming patients.

External marketing encompasses a number of methods for contacting prospective patients, including radio and television spots (advertisements or public information segments), notices in telephone directories, community speaking engagements by the dentist or a designated team member, newspaper columns, participation at health fairs, press releases, or articles about the practice printed in the newspaper.

Some dental practices use outside mailing houses or independent marketing services to distribute external marketing fliers, mailing inserts, or other notices to new residents in the neighborhood. For maximum impact, mailings are selected using predetermined local zip codes within a specific radius of the practice. Some dentists also use list management services for new move-in information from local mailing services, and direct mail organizations to send get-acquainted mailings or welcome-to-the-neighborhood greetings to new residents.

Public Speaking

Public speaking is another form of external marketing often used by dentists to gain community exposure and referrals of new patients. Public speaking is an excellent opportunity for the dentist to address a particular aspect of the practice or available services, such as pit and fissure sealant, cosmetic bonding, prevention of periodontal disease, or prevention and treatment of sports-related mouth injuries.

Public speaking presentations should be geared to the specific target audience for the best effect. When addressing a parents' group, for example, the dentist may speak on development of children's teeth, the benefits of pit and fissure sealants and fluoride, chewing (spit) tobacco awareness, or preventing sports-related injuries. When speaking to a more mature target audience, the dentist may choose topics such as crown and bridge, prevention and treatment of periodontal disease, or dental implants.

Because people in the audience often have questions about specific dental procedures, the dentist can use the speaking engagement as a marketing opportunity by providing additional appointment or business cards, practice pamphlets, or other helpful handouts. Additional effective presentation and teaching tools include educational videos and personalized patient education brochures.

Tracking Marketing Results

To analyze the effectiveness of the marketing promotion or campaign, the office manager must track the results and report them periodically to the dentist and team members. The office manager can track marketing campaign results using a variety of methods. One is to simply ask all new patients, "Who may we thank for referring you to our practice?" The office manager maintains a log (either written or on the computer) that includes the patient's name, the source of the referral, and how and when the referral was acknowledged (if appropriate).

The office manager may also track results by compiling an ongoing list of the number of new patients enrolled in the practice as a result of a direct mailing to new move-ins in nearby zip codes. The office manager should also track all specific procedures completed and note increasing or decreasing trends.

For example, the office manager tracks the total number of crown and bridge units and compares the tally with the previous monthly number. If the previous monthly average was 35 units, the practice's goal was to increase this to 40 units, and the increase was to 42 units this month, the practice's monthly goal was exceeded (Figure 5-2).

Many practices include monthly or quarterly bonuses paid to staff for sequentially meeting or exceeding production goals.

Referral Source Analysis

Referrals represent a significant source of practice growth. In fact, 80 percent of new patients are referred by 20 percent of the practice's existing patient base. Many practices use *referral source analysis* as a method for

---

Sample Goal-Tracking Form

| Month | | Year | |

SERVICES:	GOAL:	# PERFORMED:
Adult Prophies	_____	_____
Amalgam Surfaces	_____	_____
Composite Bonding Surfaces	_____	_____
Crown and Bridge Units	_____	_____
Endodontic Canals	_____	_____
Quadrants of Perio Scaling	_____	_____
Veneers	_____	_____
Tooth-Whitening Arches	_____	_____

Figure 5-2.   The goal-tracking form helps the office manager monitor and analyze production goals.

monitoring the source of new patients, the number of dollars generated as a result, and increases in demand for specific types of dental procedures or services (Figure 5-3).

The office manager maintains and prints out referral source analysis reports from the computer that provide information on the source of referrals and the total fees generated as a result.

Thanking Referral Sources

Under the dentist's direction, the office manager uses the information from the referral source analysis to send thank you cards or letters to patients or professional colleagues or associates of the dentist who refer new patients to the practice.

In addition to thank you cards and letters, many practices show their appreciation for new patient referrals by sending flowers, gift certificates, or tickets to theater or local sporting events.

Using a variety of marketing strategies and campaigns, the practice can increase new patient referrals and the demand for additional services.

Referral Source Analysis

Id		Referral Source Name	Type	Current Month ...12-01-99 to 12-19-99... # New Patients	$ Fees	Year-to-Date ...01-01-99 to 12-19-99... # New Patients	$ Fees	Cumulative ... "ALL" to "ALL" ... # New Patients	$ Fees
				(Patient Referrals)					
BENNJR	0	Jeff R. Bennett	F	2	179.00	2	79.00	3	329.00
DIXOSA	0	Susan A. Dixon	E	0	0.00	6	1,630.00	10	2,167.00
FREDJW	0	Jill W. Frederick	C	1	78.00	3	152.00	3	152.00
INGAJT	0	James T. Ingalls	E	0	0.00	3	67.00	5	404.00
JOHNWA	0	William A. Johnson	E	1	95.00	3	229.00	6	1,329.00
MORRMS	0	Maria S. Moore	B	0	0.00	0	0.00	1	28.00
OLIVSW	0	Stanley W. Oliver	F	1	47.00	4	823.00	4	823.00
PRINJA	0	Jennifer A. Prince	E	0	0.00	2	1,317.00	2	1,317.00
RICOHE	0	Harold E. Rico	E	1	66.00	4	419.00	5	492.00
				(Professional Referrals)					
SMITJO	0	John Smith, M.D.	O	4	370.00	10	830.00	10	830.00
WILSSM	0	Samual M. Wilson, M.D.	O	2	185.00	5	415.00	5	415.00
				(Marketing Referrals)					
ZZ	1	Yellow Pages	Y	1	110.00	4	844.00	8	1,030.00
ZZ	6	Welcome Wagon	Y	1	98.00	3	296.00	4	326.00
		Final Totals:		14	1,228.00	49	7,101.00	66	9,642.00
		Average $ Per New Patient:			87.71		144.92		146.09

Figure 5-3. The referral source analysis form pinpoints referrals who generate new patients to the practice, as well as the corresponding production figures.

Skill-Building for Success: Student Activities

These optional activities and exercises are designed to help the student put into practice information learned in the chapter.

1. Divide into groups and choose a team leader. Within each group, every team member will be assigned to contact (call or visit) a different dental office in the area to determine what type of marketing program(s) the office does, and to request samples of their marketing materials. In a later designated class period, each team member will give a five-minute presentation of its office's marketing programs and show samples of those marketing materials. The class will discuss which marketing efforts it thinks would be most effective and give reasons why.

2. Contact direct mail companies who promote dental office marketing materials. Request a copy of their catalog(s) and samples. Bring these to the classroom and discuss ways students could use these materials in a real-life job situation working in a dental practice.

3. Invite a local dental office to send its representative (e.g., the doctor, the office manager, or the entire team) to make an office-marketing presentation to the class. Be prepared to ask questions, such as "How did you determine this was most effective for your practice?" "What would you do differently?" "What will you include in your next marketing campaign?"

Skills Mastery Assessment: Post-Test

Directions: Select the response that *best* answers each of the following questions. Only one response is correct.

1. The need for dental offices to engage in marketing campaigns has evolved due to all of the following *except:*
   a. changes in dental practice patterns
   b. an increase in the birth rate
   c. reduction of dental insurance benefits
   d. increased dental school enrollments

2. Practiced ethically, marketing concepts can be successfully used to:
   a. increase the number of new patients
   b. increase the demand for services from the existing patient base
   c. generate referrals
   d. any or all of the above

3. Marketing is the promotion of products or services available from a specific business or organization through a variety of media.
   a. True
   b. False

4. Forms of media the dental practice may use for marketing include:
   a. radio and television broadcasting
   b. billboards, newspapers, and magazines
   c. advertisements in telephone directories
   d. any or all of the above

5. Dental practices may ethically promote their services using a variety of _____ and _____ strategies.
   a. internal/external
   b. formal/informal
   c. exogenous and intravenous
   d. ethical and unethical

6. On average, U.S. dental practices spend about _____ percent of their total overhead on marketing.

   a. 5
   b. 8
   c. 10
   d. 12

7. Examples of event marketing include:

   a. patients' birthdays
   b. anniversaries with the practice
   c. patient attributes
   d. a and b only

8. Patient satisfaction may be measured through:

   a. telephone surveys
   b. face-to-face surveys with patients
   c. patient focus groups
   d. any or all of the above

9. External marketing may include target mailings to new residents in the neighborhood according to zip code numbers.

   a. True
   b. False

10. The result of any marketing promotion or campaign is incomplete without tracking the results.

    a. True
    b. False

11. Referral source analysis reports created by the office manager provide information that:

    a. pinpoints referral sources who recommend new patients
    b. reports the total fees generated from these new patients
    c. reflects the results of patient satisfaction surveys
    d. all of the above

12. In addition to sending thank-you cards and letters, some practices show their appreciation for new patient referrals with:
    a. complementary dinners
    b. flowers sent to the referrer's place of business
    c. tickets to the theater or local sporting events
    d. all of the above

13. The key elements to a successful dental marketing campaign include all of the following *except:*
    a. creating a need
    b. demonstrating expertise
    c. emphasizing overall expense
    d. offering convenience

14. Psychological correlation to elevated self-esteem, increased self-confidence, and a youthful appearance or preservation of the patient's natural smile are marketing benefits that are often used to create a need for services in the mind of the patient.
    a. True
    b. False

15. To be measurable, a goal must be definable.
    a. True
    b. False

16. The dentist recently purchased a new laser and wants to market the benefits of laser treatment to patients. Which of the following represents the *best* measurable goal that can be tracked?
    a. To inform and educate our patients about the benefits of laser treatment.
    b. To inform and educate our patients about the benefits of laser treatment and to schedule 10 laser appointments per month during the first quarter of the year.
    c. To compare our laser treatment figures to those of another practice in the building.
    d. all of the above

References

Baum, N. (1992). *Marketing your clinical practice ethically, effectively, economically.* Gaithersburg, MD: Aspen Publishers, Inc.

Bernstein, A. (1988). *The health professional's marketing handbook.* Chicago: Year Book Medical Publishers, Inc..

Blair/McGill Advisory. (1996, September).

Brown, S. (1986). *Marketing strategies for physicians: A guide to practice growth.* Oradell, NJ: Medical Economics.

Brown, S. (1993). *Patient satisfaction pays: Quality service for practice success.* Gaithersburg, MD: Aspen Publishers, Inc.

Hutcheson, C. (1997, November/December). *Are we dental assistants marketing and promoting our practices? The Dental Assistant, Journal of the American Dental Assistants Association.*

Jameson, C. (1994). *Great communication = great production.* Tulsa, OK: PennWell Publishing Company.

Leebov, W. (1990). *Patient satisfaction: A guide to practice enhancement.* Oradell, NJ: Medical Economics.

Practice Outlook, Phoenix, AZ.

Stallard, R. (1986). *Handbook of dental marketing: Ideas and techniques that work.* Tulsa, OK: Pennwell Publishing Company.

The complete dental marketing handbook, ©Healthcare Management Services: NY. (1988). Phoenix, AZ: SmartPractice.

The Ultimate Computer System Illustration Guide. Phoenix, AZ: Practice Outlook®, Inc.

Wilson, J. (1991). *Word-of-mouth marketing.* New York: John Wiley & Sons, Inc.

Chapter 6

Printed Communications

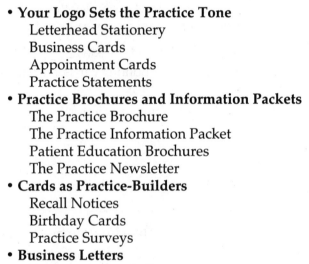

- **Your Logo Sets the Practice Tone**
  Letterhead Stationery
  Business Cards
  Appointment Cards
  Practice Statements
- **Practice Brochures and Information Packets**
  The Practice Brochure
  The Practice Information Packet
  Patient Education Brochures
  The Practice Newsletter
- **Cards as Practice-Builders**
  Recall Notices
  Birthday Cards
  Practice Surveys
- **Business Letters**
  Business Letter Styles
  Welcome to the Practice Letter
  Thank You for the Referral Letter
- **Other Printed Communications from the Practice**

Learning Objectives

Upon completion of this chapter, the student will achieve an 80 percent or higher score on the Skills Mastery Assessment Post-Test *covering the following material.*

1. Describe the importance of a logo in practice identity.

2. List the components of letterhead stationery.

3. Describe the reasons for all staff members to have practice business cards.

4. List the necessary information contained on an appointment card.

5. List the components of a practice statement.

6. Describe the importance of a practice brochure and introductory information packet.

7. List the ways patient education brochures are used effectively in practice communications.

8. Describe important components of a practice newsletter and the role of the office manager in newsletter organization and production.

9. Describe the importance of recall cards in retaining patients.

10. Describe how birthday cards and other holiday cards are used as an effective marketing tool in the dental office.

11. List the components of a well-written business letter.

Key Terms

appointment card	patient education brochures
business card	practice brochure
information packet	practice survey
letterhead stationery	recall card
logo	referral(s)
newsletter	statement
on-line	

The dental office manager is the primary communications director for the practice. As such, it is her or his responsibility to see that all communications, whether printed, electronic, or verbal, are in keeping with the doctor's standards and the philosophy of the practice. This chapter addresses the primary components of printed communications arising from the dental office.

Your Logo Sets the Practice Tone

A **logo** is a design or symbol that represents a business, or in this case, a dental practice. The practice logo may consist of a visual graphic (picture or symbol), letters, words, the name of the practice or the doctor's name, or all of these elements.

Great care and thought must be used when designing or changing a practice logo, as this is the symbol patients, other professionals, and members of the community recognize as representing the dentist and the office.

A logo reflects the tone or philosophy of the practice, and may be as simple as a single tooth or letter and may be friendly and casual in nature. The logo may also reflect the type of the practice (general or specialty) and specific services offered (Figure 6-1).

Once established, the logo appears on all printed communications of the practice. These may include, but are not limited to, stationery, business cards, appointment cards, recall notices, monthly statements, uniforms and scrubs, checks, envelopes, practice brochures, information packets, newsletters, recall cards, and other imprinted giveaways.

Letterhead Stationery

Office **letterhead stationery** is a key component in printed communications to patients, other doctors' offices, and professional contacts. It contains all pertinent information required to contact the doctor or the practice, including the name of the practice (if used), the doctor's name, credentials and other initials (DDS, DMD, PC, FAGD), the office address, telephone number, and fax number. If the office is **on-line,** it may also contain the practice's *e-mail address* or *website address.*

A stationery package includes standard sized business paper (8 1/2" x 11") with matching envelopes. It may also include additional blank pages (for second pages of letters), smaller note paper (called "monarch" size)

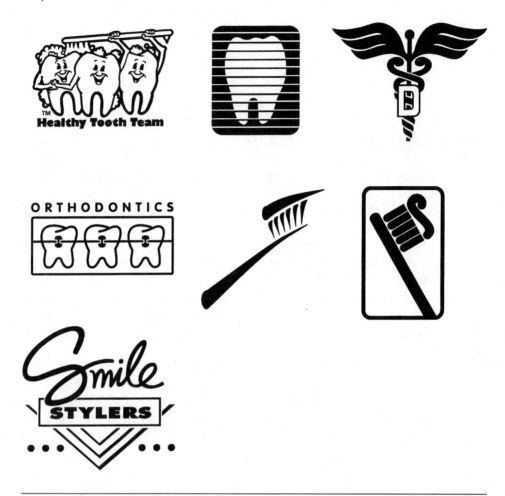

Figure 6-1. Sample dental logos. *(reprinted courtesy ©SmartPractice, Inc. Phoenix, AZ. All rights reserved. To order call 800-522-0800.)*

with matching envelopes, and/or note pads. All pieces of letterhead stationery are printed with identical practice information and the logo.

Many dentists also have their prescription pads printed with the letterhead stationery and logo and other pertinent information required for writing prescriptions. Many include the dentist's *DEA* narcotics license number on their prescription pads (Figure 6-2).

Telephone: (612) 545-3200   DEA #AP 1234567

DR. ARTHUR J. PETTERSON, P.C.

7801 Winpark Drive   Minneapolis, MN 55427

Name_____ Date_____

Address_____

℞

Figure 6-2. Sample prescription pad. *(reprinted courtesy Medical Arts Press, Minneapolis, MN.)*

Business Cards

The **business card** is also a key component of the practice's printed communications. The business card is essentially a marketing device that contains all of the information found on the letterhead stationery in a condensed size.

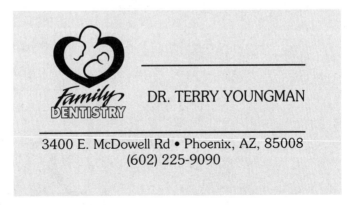

DR. TERRY YOUNGMAN

Family DENTISTRY

3400 E. McDowell Rd • Phoenix, AZ, 85008
(602) 225-9090

Figure 6-3. Sample business card. *(reprinted courtesy ©SmartPractice, Inc. Phoenix, AZ. All rights reserved. To order call 800-522-0800.*

Many practices offer their business cards prepunched to be inserted into a desktop *Rolodex*™ card holder or magnetized for easy reference (Figure 6-3).

Business cards are given out to promote the practice and as a convenient means for patients of record, prospective patients or other professionals to contact the office.

Many practices also provide individual business cards for all of their staff members. Individual business cards promote self-esteem and provide staff members the opportunity to promote the practice to prospective patients. Business cards also encourage patients to call following appointments with treatment questions or concerns.

Appointment Cards

The primary purpose of the **appointment card** is a courtesy to remind patients of their next dental visit. Typically, the appointment card contains the business card information on one side and the specifics of the appointment on the reverse. Like a business card, the appointment card provides all the information necessary to contact the office.

Some practices also have self-adhesive appointment cards with a peel-off back that may be attached to a desk or wall calendar as a reminder of an appointment (Figure 6-4).

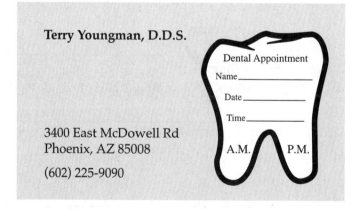

Figure 6-4.   Sample appointment card. *(reprinted courtesy ©SmartPractice, Inc. Phoenix, AZ. All rights reserved. To order call 800-522-0800.)*

Specific appointment information includes the patient's name, the day of the month, the day of the week, and the date and time. In a practice with multiple dentists, the appointment card may also indicate the name of the specific doctor (or hygienist) who will be treating the patient.

Most appointment cards also contain an office policy statement requesting the patient contact the office 24 hours in advance if a change of appointment is necessary. This is a courtesy to the office that prevents lost production time due to *disappointments* or broken appointments. It is the policy of some practices to assess a minimum charge for broken appointments.

Practice Statements

The practice **statement** is the primary means by which a practice receives compensation from patients for services provided. Thus, statements are an important printed communication from the practice.

The practice statement contains all information provided on the office letterhead. It also contains the name of the patient, party responsible (if - different), the type of service(s) rendered, the fee(s) for service(s) rendered, the amount(s) paid, the age of the account (how many days the balance has been owed to the practice), and the balance due. (See *Chapter 12, Managing Accounts Receivable*, for additional information on patient statements.)

The practice statement may also be used to communicate information on new services available, extended office hours, holiday greetings, or to introduce new staff members.

Practice Brochures and Information Packets

Disseminating information about the office may also be done with practice brochures, information packets, patient education brochures, and newsletters.

The Practice Brochure

A **practice brochure** (sometimes referred to as a "Welcome to the Practice" brochure) introduces the practice philosophy and policies to new patients. A practice brochure can:

- increase recognition of the practice name among existing and prospective patients

- communicate the practice's mission statement and philosophy
- provide information about the practice, including the location, office hours, payment plans, acceptance of insurance and other third-party payment systems, and the types of services available to accommodate patients
- indicate education and level of experience of the dentist, hygienist, dental assistant, office manager, and receptionist

The practice brochure can be used:

- as a marketing piece to attract new patients
- to reinforce the practice to patients of record
- as a referral communication device to other professionals

The Practice Information Packet

The practice **information packet** provides a number of pieces of information about the practice. It is often used in conjunction with a practice brochure to describe, in greater detail, amenities, services, and policies of the office such as a children's play area, handicapped access ramps and parking, and referral to specialists.

The practice information packet may additionally contain:

- an enlarged map inset and printed directions to the office
- a description of public transportation and parking amenities
- the doctor's educational training and background, area(s) of expertise, a brief history of the practice, and the doctor's personal philosophy and hobbies or outside interests
- an introduction of staff members and their respective roles in the practice
- appointment and cancellation policies
- financial policies and general fee information
- information for new patients about what to expect
- the individualized types of services offered
- requests for referrals

Patient Education Brochures

Patient education brochures help inform patients about oral conditions and the need for preventive, restorative, postoperative, or corrective treatment. They save valuable chairside time explaining procedures and reinforcing information given by the doctor during chairside consultations or in formal case presentations.

Patient education brochures are available in a wide variety of topics and help answer patients' most commonly asked prevention and treatment questions. Patient education brochures also serve as a reminder to the patient when explaining proposed treatment to a family member following the conclusion of the appointment.

Patient education brochures should be imprinted or rubber ink stamped with the office name or doctor's name, address, and telephone number. This information readily assists patients who wish to call the office with additional questions about treatment or postoperative care.

Many offices have a display rack featuring a variety of patient education printed materials in their reception areas. These may be purchased from the American Dental Association (ADA) or a variety of dental stationery companies.

The Practice Newsletter

Many practices send out a **newsletter** to households of patients of record and to referring colleagues. The office newsletter communicates information about the practice and the services it provides. The newsletter may also profile interesting developments in dental techniques and treatments and offer professional advice to patients.

A newsletter may be prepared by the doctor and staff or may be prepared by an outside professional newsletter service. Most often, it is the office manager's responsibility to prepare the production schedule and arrange for content of the newsletter, ensure that it is printed, the labels are printed, and that it is mailed out in a timely manner.

Newsletter content is most often determined by specific columns or topics of interest, such as a letter from the doctor, clinical or treatment updates, puzzles, games, healthful recipes, staff news, or practice changes. The newsletter may also be used to announce specific practice events or promotions (such as a smile contest), share news of the doctor and staff visiting a local school, or to promote oral hygiene and regular dental visits at a local health fair, as well as inform readers of postgraduate and / or continuing education courses completed by the doctor and / or staff.

Each newsletter issue may also carry a seasonal theme or event, such as "back-to-school checkup time" or "sealed with a smile" to promote pit and fissure sealants. For additional information on practice newsletters, refer to *Chapter 4, The Dental Office Manager as Patient Relations Specialist.* (Figure 6-5).

Cards as Practice-Builders

Many practices also use cards to communicate with patients. The most commonly sent cards include recall notices, birthday cards, and anniversary cards.

Recall Notices

Returning patients, called "recall patients," represent a significant lifeline to the practice. A **recall card** is a printed reminder of the need for a return visit for preventive dental care, usually issued every six months, although some periodontal patients may require three-month recall appointments.

Many practices preappoint recall patients and then mail the recall card one to two weeks prior to the appointment. Other practices prefer to wait until a patient is due for a recall appointment and contact patients with a phone call or send a printed recall reminder card (Figure 6-6). (See *Chapter 11, Scheduling to Optimize Practice Efficiency,* for further information on recall scheduling.)

Birthday Cards

Many practices include date of birth in individual patient's data files. In recording this information for medical and insurance purposes, many practices have made a custom of printing out a monthly list of patients' birthdays and sending automated birthday cards. Some practices send cards or letters for special occasions, such as Thanksgiving, as an alternative holiday greeting (Figure 6-7).

Newsletter Pointers for The Busy Practice

Following are helpful guidelines when planning a practice newsletter:

- **Plan ahead** – start organizing two to three months before the first mail date; set a production schedule for one year in advance.
- **Organize your thoughts** – determine the most important topics; start a file on newsletter topics and ideas. Start collecting samples of other professional newsletters that have appeal.
- **Determine the frequency of circulation** – most practices mail on a quarterly (seasonal) basis.
- **Determine content and format** – 8 1/2" x 11" printed on both sides (folded) and 11" x 17" printed on both sides (folded twice) are the most popular sizes.
- **Allocate the space for specific columns/topics in the layout** – for example, 25 percent for the doctor's letter; 10 percent for staff news; 25 percent for clinical updates and treatment techniques; 5 percent for puzzles and recipes; 20 percent for the mailing panel and address label; and 15 percent for the masthead and photos.
- **Get help from the experts if you need it** – enlist the assistance of a graphic artist or a professional copywriter, if necessary. Ask at least two other people to proofread the copy before you print the newsletter.
- **Write in personal terms** – use "you" and "your" and include patients' names (with permission). Patients like to see their names in print.
- **Emphasize total quality care and service** – include the name of a staff member and the office telephone number for readers to contact with questions or comments.
- **Solicit feedback** – ask patients for their reactions to the newsletter. Ask how you could make subsequent issues even better. Reward the best suggestions for practice improvements or enhancements and print the names of patients who submit them.
- **Monitor readership** – include an action/response device in the newsletter (e.g., a coupon, a contest, a free toothbrush, free lunch drawing, etc.) and have patients bring it in at their next appointment. This is also an excellent way to determine who actually reads the newsletter.

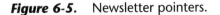

Figure 6-5.   Newsletter pointers.

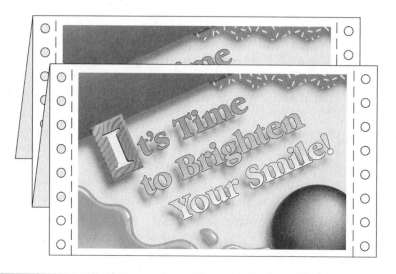

Figure 6-6. Sample recall card. *(reprinted courtesy ©SmartPractice, Inc. Phoenix, AZ. All rights reserved. To order call 800-522-0800.)*

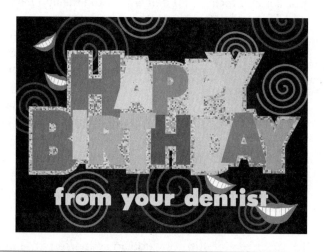

Figure 6-7. Sample birthday card. *(reprinted courtesy ©SmartPractice, Inc. Phoenix, AZ. All rights reserved. To order call 800-522-0800.)*

Practice Surveys

The **practice survey** (sometimes referred to as a patient satisfaction survey) is another way to communicate with patients. This type of written communication enables the practice to improve existing services and amenities, extend office hours, and make improvements in communications or connections with patients. The practice survey may be designed to be completed *anonymously* by the patient and either placed into a survey box located in the reception area or mailed back to the practice with a stamped, self-addressed return envelope (Figure 6-8).

Practice surveys are a key measure in assessing patients' levels of satisfaction with service and treatment. They provide information in areas where improvements can be made in efficiency, delivery of services, and courtesy.

Business Letters

The responsibility for developing well-written business letters most often belongs to the office manager. A well-written letter includes a structure that conveys a message with clarity and professionalism.

A business letter contains the following components:

- the date
- the address and salutation

Your Opinion Matters to Us

Please tell us how we're doing:

	Excellent	Good	Fair	Poor
Courtesy of Staff	❏	❏	❏	❏
Convenience of Office Hours	❏	❏	❏	❏
Waiting Room Time	❏	❏	❏	❏
Comfort During Treatment	❏	❏	❏	❏
Overall Visit	❏	❏	❏	❏
Comments				

#IN-0004 © SmartPractice

Figure 6-8. Sample patient satisfaction questionnaire *(reprinted courtesy ©SmartPractice, Inc. Phoenix, AZ. All rights reserved. To order call 800-522-0800.)*

- the body copy
- the close
- the postscript (optional)
- the enclosure (optional)

Business Letter Styles

Business letters are written in different *styles,* depending upon the type of letter and the doctor's preference.

Full block style – there are no indentations; all copy begins at the left margin.

Block I style – the inside address is flush with the left margin; the date and complimentary close are slightly off center page and aligned with each other.

Block II style – this style uses block form with no indentations or punctuation after the salutation or complimentary close.

Semi-block style – the inside address is blocked; the first line of each paragraph is indented; the date and complimentary close are slightly to the right of center page. The letter contains a subject page.

Official style – there is no subject line; each paragraph is indented. The date and complimentary close are at the center of the page.

AMS simplified style – this style saves time; it contains no salutation or complimentary close. There are no indentations.

Welcome to the Practice Letter

Because new patients are a vital key to continued practice growth, one of the most common types of letters written to patients is a welcome to the practice letter (Figure 6-9).

Thank You for the Referral Letter

Because **referrals** represent a significant form of practice-building for all professionals, another important letter from the dental office to

Date, Year

Mrs. Janice Larson
793 West Wishing Well Lane
Morrison, UT 84076

Dear Mrs. Larson:

Thank you for choosing us as your dental team. We are delighted to welcome you to our family dental practice.

We are committed to excellence and providing you the finest quality dental care available. Our goal is to help you attain and keep a beautiful smile for a lifetime.

We are looking forward to your first visit on Monday, April 7th, at 10:00 a.m. Please bring any insurance forms or other pertinent information with you at that time.

Your appointment will take approximately 45 minutes. Thank you, again, for choosing us as your dental health care providers.

Sincerely,

Philip R. Richardson, DDS

P.S. Enclosed is a brochure to acquaint you with the office. If you have any questions about your first visit or need directions, please call Vicky at 555-8990.

Figure 6-9. Sample welcome new patient letter.

another practitioner or a patient is a "thank you for the referral" letter. A referral is a recommendation made by one person to another (Figure 6-10).

Date, Year

Mr. Dale M. Everett
156 Mountain View Road, C-3
Santa Fe, NM 87115

Dear Mr. Everett:

You recently referred April Russell to our office. Referrals from friends of the practice like you are the nicest compliment we could receive.

We appreciate your loyalty and confidence in us. It's our pleasure to extend the same care and quality of treatment to friends of yours.

Thank you for placing your confidence in us.

Sincerely,

Dr. Martha McPherson Taylor and Staff

P.S. Enclosed are some additional business cards. Please pass them on to a friend or colleague who may be looking for a new dentist.

Figure 6-10. Sample thank you for the referral letter.

Other Printed Communications from the Practice

The practice may use additional printed communications for promotional efforts to patients of record and to prospective patients. These include, but are not limited to, imprinted practice giveaways such as pens, pencils, toothbrushes, tote bags, magnets, key chains, and mugs. The purpose of imprinted practice giveaways is to generate referrals and to make it easy for patients to contact the office by having the doctor's name and telephone number readily available.

Skill-Building for Success: Student Activities

These optional activities and exercises are designed to help the student put into practice information learned in the chapter.

1. You have just been hired as office manager in a busy practice. Dr. Jones is taking in a new partner (Dr. Brown) and wants you to write the copy for a practice brochure, introducing the new partner and the practice's policies. Review the text copy for ideas, then make up the office address, telephone number, office hours, and policies. (Approximate working time: 45-60 minutes)

2. Dr. Garcia just completed an extensive crown and bridge case on Mrs. Dorothy Collins, who resides at 514 Willow Street, Chicago, IL 60611. He has asked you to write a letter thanking her for being an exceptionally cooperative patient and complimenting her on her new smile. He would like you to include a postscript offering to accept her friends, family members, or coworkers as patients, should they be looking for a new dentist.

(Approximate working time: 20–30 minutes)

Skills Mastery Assessment: Post-Test

Directions: Select the response that *best* answers each of the following questions. Only one response is correct.

1. The practice logo may consist of:
   a. a visual graphic
   b. letters and words
   c. the name of the practice or the doctor's name
   d. all of these elements

2. The practice logo:
   a. is the symbol patients, professionals, and members of the community come to recognize as representing the dentist
   b. reflects the mood or philosophy of the office
   c. reflects the type of the practice
   d. all of the above

3. Patient education brochures:
   a. inform patients about oral conditions and the need for specific types of treatment
   b. reinforce the information given by the doctor during chairside consultations or in formal case presentations
   c. save valuable chairside time taken to explain procedures
   d. all of the above

4. Which of the following is *not* a feature of a practice survey?
   a. a way to communicate with patients
   b. a way to improve existing services and amenities
   c. a method of collecting overdue accounts
   d. a way to make improvements in communication

5. For best results, a practice survey must always be done anonymously.
   a. True
   b. False

6. Which of the following is *not* a necessary component of a well-written business letter?
   a. the enclosure
   b. today's date
   c. address and salutation
   d. body copy

7. The practice survey is a key measure in assessing patients' levels of satisfaction with service and treatment.
   a. True
   b. False

8. _____ is the primary communications director for the practice.
   a. the dental hygienist
   b the dental lab technician
   c. the office manager
   d. the dental supply representative

9. The practice's letterhead stationery features:
   a. the name of the practice
   b. the doctor's name and credentials
   c. the office address, telephone number, and fax number
   d. all of the above

10. Prescription pads printed with the letterhead and practice logo may also include:
    a. the office hours
    b. the dentist's DEA (narcotics) license number
    c. the date and time of the patient's next appointment
    d. the patient's known drug allergies

11. The practice statement contains:
    a. the name of the responsible party
    b. the fee(s) for service(s) rendered
    c. the amount(s) paid
    d. all of the above

12. A letter written in full block style has:

    a. no indentations
    b. all copy beginning at the left margin
    c. the date and complimentary close slightly off center page
    d. a and b only

13. Most appointment cards contain an office policy statement requesting the patient contact the office 24 hours in advance if a change of appointment is necessary. This:

    a. is a courtesy to the office
    b. prevents lost production time due to *disappointments* or broken appointments
    c. may result in assessment of a broken appointment charge to the patient
    d. all of the above

14. The practice statement may be used to communicate:

    a. information on new services available
    b. extended office hours and holiday greetings
    c. introduction of new staff members
    d. all of the above

References

Dietz, E. *Newsletter pointers for the busy practice.* [Seminar Handout]. Phoenix, AZ: SmartPractice.

How to develop a practice brochure. (1992). (ADA Marketing Handbook Series). Chicago: American Dental Association.

Jameson, C. (1994). Great communication = great production. Tulsa, OK: PennWell Publishing Company.

Wiles, C., & Dietz, E. (1989). *The complete dental letter handbook: Your fingertip resource for practice communications.* Phoenix, AZ: Semantodontics.

Chapter 7

Business Office Equipment: Hub of the Practice

- **Practice Communication Equipment**
- **The Telephone**
    Telephone Features
    Callers "On-hold"
    Speaker
    Headphones
    The Conference Call
    Conference Call Etiquette
    Voice Mail and Voice Messaging
    Answering Service
    Tone of Service
    Telephone Courtesy
    Pager
- **Fax Machine**
- **Photocopy Machine**
- **The Practice Computer**
- **Hardware**
    Input Devices
    CPU (Central Processing Unit)/System Unit
    Secondary Storage
    Output Devices
- **Software Functions**
    Selecting Software
    Software Extensions

Learning Objectives

Upon completion of this chapter, the student will achieve an 80 percent or higher score on the Skills Mastery Assessment Post-Test *covering the following material.*

1. Describe the importance of the telephone as the primary communication contact between patients and the office.
2. Be familiar with the different types of telephone messaging systems, on-hold systems, and conference calling.
3. Discuss the elements and uses of a fax machine and pager in a typical practice.
4. Differentiate between computer hardware and software components and describe their functions.
5. List the features of a dental software system and discuss software extensions.

Key Terms

byte	output device(s)
CPU (Central Processing Unit)	pager
disk	software
hardware	voice mail
input device(s)	voice messaging

Practice Communication Equipment

Running a modern dental practice efficiently requires the same proficiency and high-tech equipment as other fast-paced for-profit businesses. The office manager may already be familiar with many of the basic components of an automated practice; however, constant upgrading of applications requires continuous learning and retraining.

The Telephone

The telephone is the "voice" of the practice. It represents the office's personality to the community and is the first and primary point of contact with patients in their introduction to the practice.

The minimum for most dental practices is two lines into the main number. Many offices have at least two incoming lines for the practice and often a third, for personal calls, which rings into the dentist's private office. Occasionally, a fourth line is provided for outbound calls. Some practices have a call-waiting or call-forwarding feature that allows messages to be picked up from another number.

Most commonly the telephone at the front desk is wired for the office manager to receive all incoming calls, including personal calls for the dentist. The line on which a specific call is received, usually associated with a light on the key panel, alerts the office manger to the incoming line to allow him or her to extend the proper greeting.

Telephone Features

Many dental practices use a telephone system with some form of *caller I.D. (identification)*. This is a digital panel that displays the number of the calling party. Most dental office phones also feature a *hold button*, which plays music from a radio station, prerecorded music, or a specially recorded message for the holding caller.

Callers "On-hold"

"On-hold" music or prerecorded messages are provided by a digitalized internal system created by a specialty marketing firm. Callers hear information about elective procedures performed by the practice, such as cosmetic dentistry or passive bleaching, or treatment or technological updates. If the practice sponsors patient-appreciation events, the upcoming events can be recorded by the office manager as part of the "on-hold" message.

Alternatively, some practices program music without voice-overs onto their "on-hold" recording. Other practices use technology that transfers callers on hold directly to the ongoing broadcast of a local radio station.

Speaker

Many dental office phones feature a built-in speaker that allows the user to engage in a conversation without having to pick up the receiver. Another benefit of a built-in speaker is to enable a group of people in the same room to hold a conference call using only one telephone.

Headphones

Most sophisticated dental office telephones are adaptable for a jack and headphones. Some dental office managers prefer to wear a headset for greater efficiency when both hands are free for data entry and filing, appointment scheduling and confirmation, and to maintain a more comfortable posture.

The Conference Call

Another popular option of the dental office telephone is conference calling capability, which allows the user to connect additional lines to an existing line.

For better service with larger conferences (more than three parties on each end) it becomes necessary to schedule a "dial-in" or "operator-dialed" call. The office manager does this by calling the long distance carrier that services the practice.

The telephone company representative creates a *voice bridge* that permits a number of dialers to call a toll-free number, enter an *access code*, and join the conference call. The dental office's account is billed for the call. The conference call has a different access code.

A second option is for the office manager to have the operator dial the conference call. In this process, the long-distance operator dials each of the parties to the call and adds them to the conference at the appointed time.

If the practice phone system has a built-in conferencing feature, the office manager presses the *conference* button rather than the *hold* button, dials a second party, presses the conference button a second time enabling the new party to talk to the first person who was called as well as to the originator, in a three-way conversation.

This conference call principle also works with inbound calls. If a caller on the second line wishes to join the conversation on the first line, the office manager presses the *conference* button to place the first line on hold, opens the second line, and presses *conference* again. This joins the two incoming callers on a common *bridge* that allows all of the other callers to communicate with each other in conference.

If the practice works closely with dental specialists, the conference call is often the most effective way to handle patient referrals or consultations.

Conference Call Etiquette

The appropriate etiquette for a conference call is for the office manager to introduce everyone participating. For example, the office manager says, "Hello, Jayne. This is Shannon from Dr. James Olsen's office. Also on the line are Dr. Olsen, Charlyn Roberts, his hygienist, and our patient, Daniel Smith, whom we have referred to Dr. Donaldson for periodontal surgery."

If the office manager has not yet connected the patient, she should announce her intention to do so. For example, "If there are no questions, I would like to add Mr. Smith to the line for directions to your office and questions about his surgery." If there are no questions, the office manager can say, "I'll leave the line for a brief moment while I add Mr. Smith."

When the patient answers, the office manager tells him, "Mr. Smith, I have Dr. Olsen, Dr. Donaldson, his scheduler, Jayne, and Dr. Olsen's hygienist, Charlyn, holding on a conference call. Would you like to join us for directions to Dr. Donaldson's office and a brief review on your scheduled surgery?"

The office manager then presses the conference button again, adding the second line to the conference call. She announces that Mr. Smith has joined her on the line. The specialist's scheduler can then respond by saying, "Hello, Shannon, Dr. Olsen, Charlyn, and Mr. Smith. Thank you for calling. Dr. Donaldson is standing by to join us. May I place you on hold a moment while I add him to our conference?"

Dr. Donaldson then joins the call from his desk and says "Hello, Mr. Smith, Dr. Olsen, Shannon, and Charlyn. Jayne Howard, who will be scheduling Mr. Smith's appointment, is with me on the line. Mr. Smith, I have your radiographs on my viewbox and Dr. Olsen's recommendations here in front of me on my desk. Do you have any questions about your surgery?"

If it becomes necessary or convenient for one of the parties to disconnect, it is courteous to inform the others. The office manager can say,

"Excuse me, Dr. Olsen and Dr. Donaldson, I'm going to say good-bye and complete Mr. Smith's paperwork if there are no further issues regarding the appointment time or place. Mr. Smith, I will be following up with Jayne and she will take care of your insurance claim for the surgery." This excuses the others from trying to include the office manager in the discussion later, to be answered only by silence.

Voice Mail and Voice Messaging

Another telephone feature in many dental offices is **voice mail**, a recorded message service that intercepts the line after a set number of rings and asks the caller to leave a message. With a basic voice mail system the call will not be answered if the line is busy.

More sophisticated than voice mail is **voice messaging**. With this capability, if a caller dials the office while both lines are busy, the system automatically answers the call with a recorded message rather than transmitting a busy signal. The system announces that the call is being answered by the messaging system, the party (mentioned by name) is unavailable to take the call at the moment, but will return the call as soon as possible.

The recorded message then invites the caller to leave a phone number and detailed message for that purpose. This capability can be further enhanced by offering a delayed live response, if the caller prefers to hold for an available line or to press zero for operator assistance.

If the practice offers this option, it can also be programmed to play the "on-hold" message, a custom digitalized recording that describes the practice, information regarding office hours or location, or an interesting aspect of dentistry, often recorded over background music.

Answering Service

Many dental practices engage a professional answering service to ensure all emergencies are addressed according to policy. The answering service personnel can be scripted to manage after-hours or "roll over" calls in a manner consistent with specific circumstances.

Usually the office phone can be programmed to "roll over" or forward callers to the answering service if the office manager chooses. For example, during attendance at seminars or conventions, when a list of alternate care providers needs to be consulted in special cases, will be handled differently from calls that come in during the lunch hour.

The answering service handles calls differently when the dentist is out ill from those when the practice receives an unusually heavy volume of calls. Some offices exercise the maximum amount of control over varying situations by employing an answering service as back-up to the electronic answering options of the phone system. Depending upon the complexity of the options available on the office phone, it may be necessary for the office manager to spend some time examining the instructions, programming the appropriate functions, and practicing the accurate execution of all the system features.

The credibility and professionalism of the practice is jeopardized if the office manager accidentally disconnects parties to a conference call, connects callers to the wrong dentist, or answers multiple lines with the wrong greeting. These errors can be avoided by studying the system and practicing the function commands ahead of time.

Tone of Service

The wise office manager knows that a professional, courteous, pleasant telephone manner is worth measurable revenue and public relations value to the practice. Some consultants call these qualities *tone of service,* a phrase that encompasses timely resolution of all the caller's issues, accuracy of all information dispensed to callers, and personality traits projected to callers, such as friendliness, helpfulness, concern, and patience. Good grammar and diction are also essential.

Some office managers "shop" their offices regularly by asking other professionals to call their practice anonymously to critique the quality of the phone response. It is every team member's responsibility to maintain the highest possible standards of practice communication and patient education. Much of this standard is portrayed via phone contacts (Figure 7-1).

Telephone Courtesy

As with all forms of communication, extreme courtesy must be exercised by the office manager when talking with patients and other callers. The office manager should answer the phone with a greeting specified by the

---

Sample Telephone Checklist

☐ Greet caller appropriately and pleasantly

☐ Remain patient and sympathetic toward confused caller

☐ Handle refusal to quote fees with positive phrases

☐ Sell caller on diagnostic consultation

☐ Handle caller who owes money with positive phrases

☐ Remain calm and professional with abusive caller

☐ Resolve complicated scheduling problems quickly

☐ Convert angry caller to happy patient

☐ Invite prospective patients to visit the practice for a complimentary tour

☐ Politely discourage suspected drug abusers from attempting to obtain narcotic prescriptions

☐ Avoid the temptation to diagnose over the phone

☐ Always let the caller hang up first

Figure 7-1.   Sample telephone checklist.

doctor, such as, "Good morning/good afternoon, Dr. Marks' office, this is Mary, how may I assist you?"

The conclusion of the telephone call must also follow the doctor's required close, such as, "Thank you for calling, Mrs. Jackson." When the office manager initiates the call she or he should conclude with "thank you." Other standard courtesies used when speaking face-to-face should also be used when speaking on the telephone (Figure 7-2).

Pager

The electronic **pager** has become an indispensable communication device in many dental offices. The pager is a cordless electronic device to which a caller directs a specific telephone number for a call to be returned. The pager activates with a buzzing sound or vibrating motion.

The doctor may use a pager to be reached during time outside of the office, for example, by the answering service to contact an emergency patient.

Telephone Courtesy Checklist

☐ Answer the telephone no later than on the second ring
☐ Always greet the caller pleasantly and identify yourself
☐ Use correct grammar
☐ Never interrupt the caller or presume the nature of the call
☐ If you must put the caller on hold, ask his or her permission first
☐ Always let the caller conclude the conversation
☐ Never hang up in anger (or frustration) or slam the receiver down
☐ Always smile when speaking on the telephone

Figure 7-2.   Telephone courtesy checklist

The office may lend pagers to parents who wish to drop off their older children for treatment while they shop or run errands. The office then pages the parent that the child's appointment is complete. Many parents appreciate this time-saving convenience.

Fax Machine

Telephone lines are also utilized for other forms of electronic communication, such as *fax (facsimile)* machines. Many documents can now be faxed, saving time and postage. Most requests for written materials can be answered by an offer to fax the information immediately.

The wise office manager familiarizes herself or himself with the office's fax machine; most models are relatively self-explanatory. Utilizing a variety of methods of programming, the machine can scan the document, dial the fax number of the recipient, and begin the transmission. Most models have a digital display that prompts the user to enter the appropriate command.

Most fax models also display the amount of memory available. They also report the status of the task, such as complete, incomplete, dialing, redialing, or receiving. A report automatically prints out if an exception or error occurs. This alerts the office manager to resend the transmission, add paper, install a new cartridge, or redial. In some cases the fax machine alerts the sender to a problem at the receiver's end, such as full memory.

The office manager should also familiarize herself with fax machine maintenance and operation principles (Figure 7-3).

Most later model fax machines can be programmed to send faxes to a multiple list of recipients that can either be entered for a one-time distribution or entered and stored as a "list" for future multiple transmissions.

Some dental computer systems are equipped with a program that faxes directly from the computer to the recipient. A specific example is a response to a patient who requests documentation on the total sum the family spent for dental services during the previous tax year. The office manager can access that report and send it to the patient's fax machine directly from the computer. Another application is recall visit information, which can be faxed to patients with access to faxed transmissions.

The office manager can command a *global fax*, which faxes a specified report or document to everyone in the program with a fax number attached to his or her personal data base.

Rules for Efficient Fax Transmissions

- Read the operating manual carefully and experiment with the features to avoid making mistakes with actual transmissions.
- Monitor the supplies regularly to avoid interruptions in service.
- Keep the paper trays filled and *never use the last toner cartridge without ordering a replacement. Note:* In an emergency, the empty toner cartridge can be removed, shaken gently to redistribute the toner material, and replaced.
- Be especially vigilant regarding patient confidentiality when using fax transmissions to communicate sensitive information. (See *Chapter 2, Legal and Ethical Issues and Responsibilities* for additional legal information regarding fax transmissions.)
- For fax transmissions that are not confidential, the office manager can save money and paper by omitting the cover page. A convenient way to identify faxes is to affix a preprinted self-adhesive note specifically made for fax transmissions to the first page. It provides spaces for the name, practice, phone and fax phone, name of the intended recipient of the fax, that person's identifying information, that person's phone and fax phone, and the number of pages being faxed.

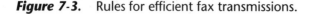

Figure 7-3.   Rules for efficient fax transmissions.

Many fax machines also have a copier feature that allows the user to make a single page photo copy.

Photocopy Machine

Most offices find the copy machine an indispensable piece of equipment. Used to duplicate patient claim forms, treatment plans, and estimates and postoperative instructions, the copy machine is designed to provide a myriad of features. These features include, but are not limited to two-sided copying, collating, sorting, stapling, reducing, and enlarging. More sophisticated copiers also have four-color capability.

As with all office equipment, the office manager should review the manufacturer's instruction and maintenance manual for operation instructions and repair information.

The Practice Computer

As in most business offices, dental offices use computers for many of their routine word-processing, billing, recall, marketing communications, and data management tasks. Following is a basic overview of computer **hardware** and **software** with which the office manager should be familiar.

Hardware

The physical or visible computing equipment is called the hardware. The hardware associated with a computer system consists of four parts: 1) the **input devices**, 2) the **CPU (Central Processing Unit)** or system unit, 3) the secondary storage devices, and 4) the **output devices**.

Input Devices

Consisting of the *keyboard* and/or *mouse* and optional *scanner*, the input devices interpret commands in a manner that allows the computer to process specific information.

The Keyboard

The main components of the keyboard are the typewriter-like keys, the numeric keypad, the function keys, and the special-purpose keys.

The *enhanced keyboard* has a row of function and special purpose keys above the regular typing keyboard, with a panel of curser control keys to the left of the numeric keypad. It is lighted, a feature which allows the user to see whether the keypad is toggled to behave as a calculator or a curser-control panel, and whether or not the *all caps* function is active.

The Mouse

The mouse is an optional feature of most computers that allows the office manager to move around the screen, avoiding repetitive keystrokes. The mouse is also used to access the tool bar at the top of the screen, a shortcut to using function keys.

The Scanner

In addition to the keyboard or mouse, some dental practices use a scanner, similar to the wand used by some retailers to read bar codes, or a larger scanner that resembles a photocopier. The scanner is capable of scanning in written material a page at a time, a photograph, or image other than text.

A scanning device often used in dental applications is the *intraoral camera*, an imaging wand that converts optical scans of the patient's oral cavity to a digital format. This can be projected onto a viewing screen for the dentist and patient to view in real time, captured as photographs, or stored on magnetic or digital disks for future reference.

Some practices also utilize more sophisticated imaging input devices that allow the system to manipulate the image for patients to view the before and after results of proposed cosmetic treatment recommendations.

CPU (Central Processing Unit)/System Unit

The CPU (Central Processing Unit) or system unit is electronic circuitry housed within the computer cabinet. This circuitry performs the memory and processing functions of computer processing. The CPU executes programs, performs calculations, and temporarily stores data and programs for those purposes.

Computer Memory

Computer *memory,* also called *primary storage,* is measured in *ROMs* or *RAMs.* ROM is the acronym for *Read Only Memory;* RAM stands for *Random Access Memory.* The ROM is built-in and is the memory that runs the applications. ROM cannot be accessed for any other purpose.

RAM is accessed temporarily during the time the system is in use, to hold the application and the data being input and processed by the word-processing program or by the spreadsheet being created. It is automatically erased when the computer is turned off. Because of this, RAM is also referred to as temporary memory.

Bytes

Computer *memory* is contained in microchips. The amount of memory of which the CPU is capable correlates to the number of microchips.

One **byte** of memory corresponds to one location, usually capable of storing one character.

A *kilobyte* equals exactly 1,024 bytes, and is often approximated as 1,000 bytes.

A *megabyte* of memory holds one million bytes; a *gigabyte* holds approximately one billion bytes. Most modern microcomputers have a minimum memory capacity of at least eight megabytes. Those with multiple gigabyte capacity are used by businesses that process millions of customer account numbers or other large commercial or scientific data bases.

Secondary Storage

Most commonly, a **disk** provides a place to store information or data that will be input for processing or installed for a specific function. This can also be used for backup functions.

Most applications such as word processing or spread sheet accounting are installed from commercial disks, which are then stored on site for future use or for backup in case the programs become damaged during use and need to be re-installed.

Secondary storage devices are also widely used for sharing data with other people using other CPUs, or as a backup filing system that ensures there are always multiple copies of valuable data. Usually there is at least one internal disk, or *hard disk,* and one or more slots or drives for external, or *floppy disks.*

The hard disk is permanent, and often consists of more than one circular metallic disk used to store data files and software programs. The hard disk is sealed to prevent foreign materials from interfering with function or causing unnecessary wear.

Modern CPUs have at least 540 megabytes of hard disk capacity. Usually they are assigned to the *C* drive and have an access arm with read-write heads that stores or retrieves information more quickly than the floppy drive(s).

Note that floppy disks (also referred to as *diskettes*) aren't actually floppy. They are 3 and 3/4", encased in plastic, with a metal shutter that moves to one side as the floppy is inserted into the disk drive, permitting access to the data. The drive also opens the small *write protection notch* on the bottom of the disk, preventing the computer from changing the information on the disk. It cannot be over-written unless the office manager uses the command to save. This prompts her or him to replace the file on the disk with the new material.

If the CPU has two floppy drives, usually the vertical one on the left is the *A* drive and the one on the right is the *B* drive. If they are arranged one above the other, the one on top is usually the *A* drive.

The system may also read *CD ROM (Compact Disk, Read-Only Memory)* disks, which use laser beams to alter the surface of the disk to store data. The CD ROM drive also uses a laser to read the pitted surface. Most CD ROM disks are 5.25" in diameter and store about 650 megabytes of data, the equivalent of 147 floppy disks.

Output Devices

Output devices comprise the equipment that translates the information from the CPU into a format that can be read by the user. The output device may be a *monitor* (screen), a *printer*, or *speaker(s)*.

Software Functions

Software refers to the instructions that direct the CPU to process information. These instructions are called *programs*. The two main groups of software are *system software* and *application software*.

System software programs, or operating systems, coordinate the hardware capabilities of the computer. They organize user commands to function, call up and start up the appropriate application software, and manage the data as it is input and output. In most cases, the system software is built in by the manufacturer and must be brand-compatible. Examples of brands may be DOS, Macintosh, OS/2, Windows, or UNIX.

Application software is usually purchased commercially, often packaged in suites containing a word-processing, spreadsheet, and slide presentation program with the addition of a form and merged database application for the professional version. Software can also be custom-written for specific applications. If the practice uses a scheduling, insurance management, practice promotion, accounts-payable tracking program, or any combination of the above, the software is custom-programmed specifically for dental practices.

Selecting Software

If the office manager is delegated to choose a dental software program, it is advisable to try out several different programs and to request a demonstration in offices that currently use them (Figure 7-4).

Questions to Ask Before Selecting Dental Software

Answers to the following questions may be helpful in making a final software selection:

- How responsive have the support personnel been?
- How long did it take for the dental team to learn to use the program?
- Which features of the program does the practice actually use as intended?
- What is the total cost to the practice?

Figure 7-4.   Questions to ask before selecting dental software.

Appointment Scheduling Software Features

Appointment scheduling is an example of a software function normally programmed by the user. Thus, the office manager must input all the relevant information about the way the practice schedules according to procedures, operators, and the dentist's preferences. The most important feature to look for in a scheduling program is a series of prompts that leads the user through this task. The software system presents a selection menu, then offers the capacity to program in additional procedures as needed. The program should be pre-calibrated for one up to six operatories, with prompts that guide the user through simple choices.

Some scheduling programs also offer a default time requirement. This allows the office manager the flexibility to allot specific times for each appointment or procedure automatically.

Another common feature is scheduling the entire treatment series or sequence. This allows the office manager to enter the treatment plan at the time the patient accepts it. The program automatically appoints the inclusive plan, including the next recall visit, and prints out a treatment calendar for the patient showing all the visits, the duration, the associated fees, and the paydown schedule including interest if any. The automatic scheduling feature can also be used to prebook hygiene appointments in advance.

In researching a dental software program, the office manager should also look for a program that automatically enters the comments onto the day's treatment notes if they are flagged as clinical.

Most scheduling programs automatically track the production of each day's patient load, in such a way that it is not visible on the printed schedule, but can be printed out separately. The production can be included on the schedule that is posted in the dentist's private office only, or in other private areas such as the instrument sterilization center.

Fee Calculations

The office manager should also ensure the program calculates fee changes based on a percentage increase over all fees, a percentage increase that affects only the procedures specified, or an item by item change of a set or variable amount. The program should reflect the percentage of the practice composed of demographics, fee-for-service procedures, or referrals. The office manager may command a series of reports reflecting how the practice would be impacted by an increase in fees. The software program can assist the office manager in sorting capabilities to reflect several different ways to recover costs, either by raising all fees by a certain percentage, or by adding a set *surcharge* to all procedures or to certain procedures.

Sort Lists

After fee schedules, the most commonly used lists are recall patients (per month), referral sources, and surgery or restorative patients, with phone numbers, for postoperative telephone courtesy calls.

Another step in which sort lists are used is to command the system to generate a merge letter and/or a mailing label for specified patients on these lists, for the purpose of informing them of recall visits or mailing a thank you letter and/or a gift for referring prospective patients to the practice.

Other lists or reports alert the doctor to the number of patients who are over 30 days, over 60 days, and over 90 days delinquent on financial arrangements. These lists are calls to action, as these patients require immediate attention to collect their outstanding balances.

Many accounts receivable programs generate a series of appropriate collection letters automatically, based on criteria entered by the office manager through a series of prompts. These are merge letters that retrieve the names and addresses of delinquent accounts directly from the *account aging* application, incorporating an electronic calendar (a timing device built into the hardware that does not rest when the computer is turned off).

The account aging capability generates a report that reflects the percentage of improvement over the accounts receivable balance for the same quarter of the previous year, over the past quarter in the current year, or grouped by term of delinquency (30, 60, or 90 days). For additional information on collections management, see *Chapter 12, Managing Accounts Receivable.*

Software Extensions

E-mail is useful for electronic newsletters, broadcasting on a web page, a bulletin board, or a chat group. Many practices utilize *Med Line,* an online research service, as a comprehensive, topical guide to on-line resources such as publications and research reports.

Modem

A *modem* is required to send or receive e-mail and to access the World Wide Web. Some CPUs have built-in modems; however, the practice may still choose to install a dedicated analog line for that purpose, keeping the telephone lines accessible to callers. The office manager should be aware that the speed of the modem determines the speed with which the computer can download information from the Web.

Skill-Building for Success: Student Activities

These optional activities and exercises are designed to help the student put into practice information learned in the chapter.

1. Divide into groups. Each group must assign a leader. The leader directs each member to contact a minimum of three area dental practices to determine the following information. What dental computer software program do you currently use? What features do you especially like about it? What additional applications or features would you want if they were available? In one week, each member of the group reports to the team leader. The team leader provides a consensus from his or her group as to the most beneficial computer programs and software applications.

2. If possible, request a computer software representative to bring a portable demonstration of dental software applications and make a presentation to the class.

3. If possible, arrange for the class to visit a dental practice in the area and request a demonstration of its computer applications.

Skills Mastery Assessment: Post-Test

Directions: Select the response that *best* answers each of the following questions. Only one response is correct.

1. Telephone automation has made personal "tone of service" less important in modern practices.
   a. True
   b. False

2. Caller I.D. provides:
   a. a video camera image of the caller
   b. camera images of both the caller and the person who answers
   c. a digital display of the number of the calling party
   d. a light which corresponds to the area code of the calling party

3. Which of the following may patients hear while on hold?
   a. digitally recorded music
   b. a local radio broadcast
   c. a recorded message
   d. any of the above or a combination

4. Due to new telephone technology, only one incoming line is now necessary regardless of the number of doctors in the practice.
   a. True
   b. False

5. Which of the following is true of telephone conferencing?
   a. three-way conferences can be accessed internally
   b. operator-dialed conferences can be pre-arranged with the long distance carrier
   c. the long distance carrier can create a voice bridge for caller-dialed conferences
   d. all of the above

6. Which of the following is a main advantage of voice messaging over voice mail?

    a. it is much less expensive and can be installed by the user
    b. it can offer a menu of tentative diagnoses and play a pre-recorded commercial message
    c. it can answer even if the line is busy and offers the option of holding for the next available line
    d. it is proven to increase collections and decrease no-shows

7. If the practice uses a sophisticated on-hold message and a voice messaging system, it is may still be economical to hire an answering service as well.

    a. True
    b. False

8. Which of the following is the main precaution regarding fax transmissions?

    a. it is very expensive
    b faxes are usually not legal documents
    c. confidentially has to be carefully guarded
    d. it is not considered "professional"

9. The pager:

    a. is a cordless electronic device to which a caller directs a specific telephone number for a call to be returned
    b. activates with a buzzing sound or vibrating motion
    c. may be used to contact the dentist during time outside of the office
    d. any or all of the above

10. Which of the following is *not* an input device?

    a. keyboard
    b. mouse
    c. printer
    d. scanner

11. What do the initials CPU stand for?

    a. computer processing unit
    b. central processing unit
    c. controlled pentium utilization
    d. computer pod unit

12. Primary storage is also called:

    a. *B* drive
    b. floppy disk
    c. read-write
    d. memory

13. Which of the following is sequenced correctly from smallest to largest?

    a. byte, megabyte, kilobyte, gigabyte
    b. megabyte, kilobyte, gigabyte, byte
    c. kilobyte, byte, megabyte, gigabyte
    d. byte, kilobyte, megabyte, gigabyte

14. What features should the office manager look for in a dental software system?

    a. it can do the required tasks with a reasonable learning effort
    b. it is compatible with other dental offices
    c. it is relatively new to the industry
    d. all of the above

15. A typical dental management software system performs all of the following applications *except:*

    a. schedules appointments
    b. deletes inactive files automatically when memory is used up
    c. creates insurance forms
    d. ages accounts and generates statements

16. Which is *not* an appropriate use of the Internet in a dental practice setting?

    a. communication with patients
    b. communication with other professionals
    c. communication with friends and relatives
    d. professional research

17. Which is/are a serious concern of all Internet users?

    a. it is very expensive
    b. files are bulky and use a lot of electricity
    c. information is often obsolete
    d. information is often not secured and cannot be kept confidential

18. The CPU:

    a. executes programs
    b. performs calculations
    c. temporarily stores data and programs
    d. all of the above

19. Even a powerful computer will download slowly from the Internet if the modem is not fast.

    a. True
    b. False

20. A small *write protection notch* on the bottom of the disk prevents the computer from changing the information on the disk. It cannot be overwritten unless the office manager uses the command to save. This prompts him or her to replace the file on the disk with the new material.

    a. True
    b. False

References

A guide to using Practice Outlook for Windows® 95. (1998). Phoenix, AZ: Practice Outlook®, Inc.

Crawford, K. (1996, Spring). Introduction to intraoral cameras. *Preview.*

Dental computer: What you don't know can cost you. (1995, May/June). *Dental Practice & Finance.*

DENTRIX™ 5.0 user's guide, a DENTRIX image user's guide.

Freyberg, B. (1996, Spring). How computers are decentralizing dental practices. *Preview.*

Golub, W. S., & Levate, C. M. (1997, August). How to profit from technology integration: An educated vision about software. *Dental Economics.*

Green, Scott R. (1997, Summer). Is your company conducting business on the information super highway? *Dental Equipment and Supplies.*

Manji, I. (1996, July/August). Beyond the bells and whistles: What high technology really delivers. *Dental Teamwork.*

Nieburger, E.J. (1996, June). Digital answering machines offer numerous advantages. *The Farran Report.*

Practice Outlook training guide and reference manual. (1998). Phoenix, AZ: Practice Outlook®, Inc.

Seltzer, S. M. (1997, December). Headsets reduce the pain of calling. *Dental Economics.*

TAB® Solutions, Palo Alto, CA.

HealthCare Communications. The Dental Mac® Series: Apple Computer Inc.

Transition to the Windows platform with SoftDent SmartData integration database by InfoSoft Inc. (1996, April). *Dental Products Report.*

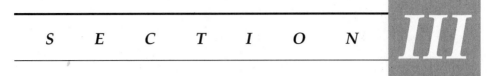

Clinical Records Management

Chapter 8

Dental Nomenclature and Related Terminology

- **Dental Arches**
  - Mandibular Arch
  - Maxillary Arch
- **Quadrants and Sextants**
- **Tooth Composition**
  - Hard Structures
  - Soft Structures
- **Anatomical Landmarks of Teeth**
- **Types and Functions of Teeth**
- **Tooth Identification: Deciduous Dentition**
- **Tooth Identification: Permanent Dentition**
- **Tooth Surfaces and Edges**
  - Mesial Surface
  - Distal Surface
  - Facial/Labial/Buccal Surface
  - Lingual Surface
  - Occlusal Surface/Incisal Edge
- **Cavity Classifications**
  - Class I
  - Class II
  - Class III
  - Class IV
  - Class V
  - Class VI

Learning Objectives

Upon completion of this chapter, the student will achieve an 80 percent or higher score on the Skills Mastery Assessment Post-Test *covering the following material.*

1. Identify the maxillary and mandibular dental arches.
2. Identify the quadrants and anterior sextants of the oral cavity.
3. List the hard and soft structures of the teeth.
4. Name all teeth comprising the primary and secondary dentition.
5. List and identify the five tooth surfaces and one edge.
6. List and define all six cavity classifications.

Key Terms

anterior	mandible
bicuspid/premolar	maxilla
buccal	mesial
canine/cuspid	molar
cementum	occlusal
deciduous/primary dentition	periodontal ligament
dentin	periodontium
distal	permanent dentition
edentulous	posterior
enamel	pulp
facial/labial	quadrants
incisal	sextants
incisor	temporomandibular joint (TMJ)
lingual	

The office manager must be thoroughly familiar with dental nomenclature (names of the teeth) and related terminology. This is essential to interpret the dentist's, hygienist's, or chairside assistant's charting and treatment-related records, and to provide patients with accurate information in pre-determining treatment costs and giving case presentations and to bill patients and third-party payors accurately for treatment performed. Knowledge of terms is also essential in educating patients about existing dental conditions and recommended treatment.

Dental Arches

The human mouth is contained in the skull (cranium) and has two jaws (arches). The *occlusal plane* is an imaginary line that distinguishes the upper and lower jaws.

Mandibular Arch

The **mandible** (jaw bone) is attached to the cranium by a moveable joint called the **temporomandibular joint (TMJ).** The mandible is the *lower* jaw.

Maxillary Arch

The **maxilla** (upper jaw) is part of the cranium and is comprised of the hard and soft palate and the maxillary teeth.

Quadrants and Sextants

The oral cavity is divided into four **quadrants** and has two **sextants.** The quadrants are determined by an imaginary horizontal line dividing the *midline* (front of the face) to designate right and left.

The four quadrants ("quad" means four) are the *maxillary right, maxillary left, mandibular right,* and *mandibular left* (Figure 8-1).

The mouth can also be divided into **anterior** (front) and **posterior** (back) teeth. The anterior sextants comprise the six anterior teeth contained in the mandible and maxilla. The posterior teeth include all remaining teeth (Figure 8-2).

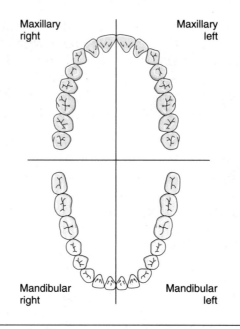

Figure 8-1.   The four quadrants of the adult dentition.

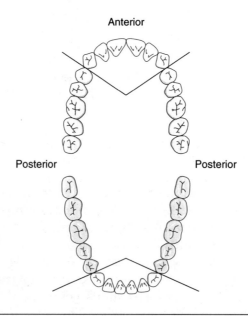

Figure 8-2.   The adult dentition showing the anterior sextant (white) and posterior (shaded) teeth.

Tooth Composition

Each tooth is imbedded in the respective jaw, attached by surrounding tissue called the **periodontium** ("perio" means around and "odont" means tooth). Each tooth is comprised of hard and soft tissues. The periodontium consists of the *gingiva* (gum tissue), *periodontal ligaments or fibers*, and the *alveolar* (bone) *process* (Figure 8-3).

Hard Structures

Hard tissues of the tooth include the **enamel, dentin**, and **cementum.**

Enamel is the hardest substance in the human body. It is composed of primarily inorganic materials and is shaped by prismatic rods. The function of enamel is to protect the tooth. Enamel ranges in color from shades of white to yellow to gray to brown.

Dentin comprises the bulk, including the crown and root portion of the tooth, and is yellower than enamel. Dentin, not enamel, determines the color of the teeth. Enamel and dentin comprise the hard tissues of the crown (portion of the tooth above the gumline). Dentin is composed of S-shaped tubules and gives shape to the tooth. It also registers sensation to pain and temperature.

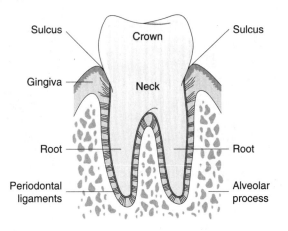

Figure 8-3. The periodontium includes the gingiva, periodontal ligaments or fibers, and the alveolar process.

Cementum is the yellowish-white outer covering of the root portion of the tooth (below the gumline). Cementum has a porous, rough, textured surface that permits the periodontal fibers to attach. Cementum can rebuild its tissue, forming *secondary cementum.* Secondary cementum growth may be stimulated by injury, abrasion, trauma, or stress (Figure 8-4).

The *roots* of the tooth have no enamel. The *crown* of the tooth has no cementum.

Soft Structures

Soft structures associated with the tooth include the **pulp** (nerve tissue) and the **periodontal ligament.** The pulp provides blood and other nutrients from the body to the tooth. It is composed of nerve, blood, and lymph. The pulp is encased in the walls of dentin and enters each tooth at a small opening in the *apex* (root tip) called the *apical foramen* (hole).

The periodontal ligament acts as a shock absorber to cushion the tooth in the socket. It also provides attachment to the jawbone. The portion of

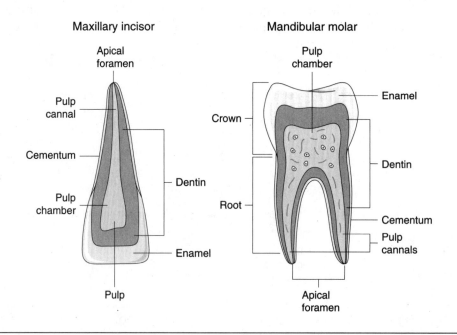

Figure 8-4. The composition of a tooth.

pulp that comprises the crown of the tooth is referred to as the *pulp chamber*. The area of the pulp that comprises the root(s) is called the *pulp canal*. Note that each root has a separate canal. Therefore, a three-rooted molar has *one* pulp chamber and *three* pulp canals.

Anatomical Landmarks of Teeth

Each tooth has specific anatomical landmarks. The most common landmarks include the following.

A *cusp* is a round mound or elevation on the working surface of a cuspid of any posterior tooth.

A *cingulum* is the lingual lobe of any anterior tooth that appears on the cervical (neck portion) one-third of the tooth.

A *lobe* is a bump arising from the tooth surface. When a lobe arises from the lingual side of the maxillary anterior teeth, it is called a *cingulum*.

A *mammelon* (also spelled mamelon) is one of three prominences of the incisal edges of newly erupted incisors.

A *ridge* is any linear elevation of a tooth surface named according to its location (e.g., "marginal" ridge).

A *marginal ridge* is a rounded border of enamel that forms the tips of the cusps of posterior teeth toward the center of occlusal surfaces.

A *transverse ridge* is formed by two triangular ridges that meet and cross the occlusal surface of any posterior tooth.

An *oblique ridge* is one that runs across the occlusal surface of maxillary molars in a diagonal direction.

A *pit* is a very small depression on a tooth surface, most often located at the end of a groove, or where two or more grooves join.

A *fissure* is a linear fault that occurs along a developmental groove between tooth lobes.

A *fossa* is an irregular depression on a tooth surface.

A *developmental groove* is a shallow groove or line on the surface of a tooth.

Types and Functions of Teeth

Teeth provide three main functions: chewing food, aiding in speech, and enhancing appearance (esthetics). The human dentition has four types of teeth.

Incisors are used for biting and cutting food. **Canines** or **cuspids** (eye teeth) are used to tear and break off food. **Bicuspids** (premolars) are used to break up and mash food. **Molars** are used to grind and pulverize food before swallowing.

Tooth Identification: Deciduous Dentition

The first set of teeth (baby teeth) is termed the **deciduous** or **primary dentition** because this set of teeth is eventually lost and replaced by the permanent (secondary) teeth.

The deciduous or primary dentition consists of 10 teeth in each arch, or five in each quadrant, making a total of 20. Starting from the midline and moving toward the back of the mouth, the teeth that comprise the deciduous dentition in each quadrant are: one *central incisor,* one *lateral* (lateral means "side") *incisor,* one *canine* (also called cuspid), and one each *first* and *second molar* (Figure 8-5).

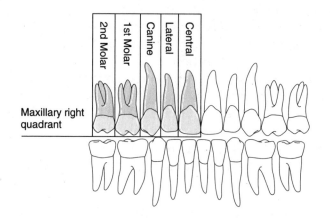

Figure 8-5.   The deciduous maxillary right quadrant with each of five teeth identified.

Tooth Identification: Permanent Dentition

The second set of teeth is termed the **permanent dentition** because these teeth comprise the final set of natural dentition. They are sometimes referred to as the secondary (second) or "succedaneous" because they succeed or follow the first or primary dentition.

The permanent dentition consists of 16 teeth in each arch, eight in each quadrant, making a total complement of 32. Starting from the midline and moving toward the back of the mouth, the eight teeth that comprise the permanent dentition in each quadrant are: one *central incisor*, one *lateral incisor*, one *canine* (also called cuspid), one each *first* and *second bicuspid* (also called premolars), and one each *first* and *second molar* and (sometimes) a *third molar* (Figure 8-6).

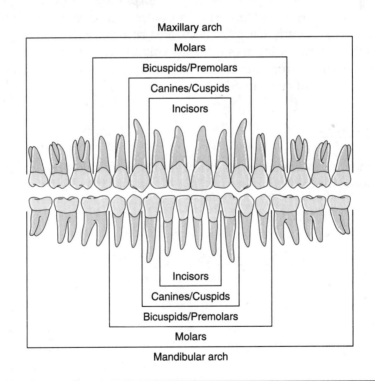

Figure 8-6. All four quadrants of the adult dentition showing the incisors, canines, bicuspids, and molars.

The permanent first and second molars are also referred to as the "six-year" and "12-year" molars because they erupt (appear) in the oral cavity at approximately those respective ages. The third molar is sometimes referred to as a "wisdom tooth" because it is the last to appear in the oral cavity and is associated with coming of age.

An adolescent who has both primary and secondary teeth in the mouth concurrently is said to have a *mixed* dentition.

A patient with no natural teeth left is said to be **edentulous**.

Tooth Surfaces and Edges

Each tooth is unique in its shape, morphology, and anatomical landmarks. Following is a description of the *surfaces* and *edges* of the human teeth. In dentistry, cavity classifications and restorative procedures are defined in terms of the surfaces or edges involved. The office manager will note that restorative procedures are billed by the *number of surfaces* treatment planned and completed.

Mesial Surface

Each tooth has a **mesial** surface. Mesial (middle) means *toward the midline* of the mouth.

Distal Surface

Each tooth has a **distal** surface. Distal (distant) means *away from the midline* of the mouth.

Facial/Labial/Buccal Surface

In the anterior sextant, each tooth has a **facial** or **labial** surface. (The terms are used interchangeably.) In the anterior teeth, this surface faces *toward the face or lips.*

In the *posterior* (back) teeth, comprised of the bicuspids and molars, the surface facing the cheeks is called the **buccal** surface (named for the buccinator or chewing muscle, adjacent to these tooth surfaces).

Lingual Surface

Each tooth has a **lingual** surface. Lingual means tongue and *faces toward the tongue.*

Occlusal Surface/Incisal Edge

In the posterior teeth, the chewing surface is referred to as the **occlusal** surface. Teeth having an occlusal surface are the premolars and molars.

In the anterior teeth there is no chewing surface, rather a *biting edge* to shear off food. This is called the **incisal** edge. Teeth having an incisal edge include the anterior sextant, the central and lateral incisors, and the canines (Figure 8-7).

Cavity Classifications

Knowledge of the specific tooth surfaces and edges is necessary to define cavity classifications. A solid understanding of cavity classifications is necessary to learn oral charting, which follows in *Chapter 9, Charting the Oral Cavity.*

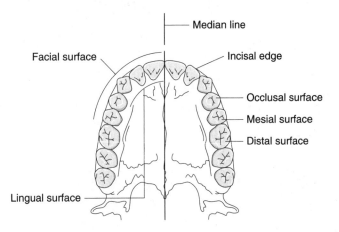

Figure 8-7.   The median line, the surfaces, and edges of the teeth depicted in the maxilla.

Class I (Anterior and Posterior Teeth)

Class I decay occurs in the developmental area of tooth, grooves, and fossae. When a developmental groove becomes faulty it is termed a *fissure;* a decayed *fossa* is called a *pit.*

Commonly referred to as "pit and fissure caries," Class I decay may occur on the occlusal surfaces of bicuspids and molars, on the buccal or lingual surfaces of molars, or on the lingual surfaces of maxillary incisors.

Class I decay is very common because decay-causing anaerobic bacteria tend to grow in the pit and fissure areas. (Pits are too small to be cleaned by a single bristle of a toothbrush.) (Figures 8-8–8-10).

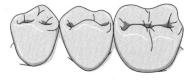

Figure 8-8.   Class I caries on occlusal surfaces of bicuspids (premolars) and molars.

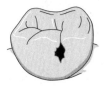

Figure 8-9.   Class I caries form on facial and lingual surfaces of molars.

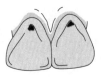

Figure 8-10.   Class I caries on lingual surfaces of maxillary incisors.

Class II (Posterior Teeth Only)

Class II decay involves the occlusal surface and either the mesial and/or distal surface of posterior teeth. Because mesial and distal surfaces are in between the teeth, they are referred to as *proximal* surfaces. This is true of all teeth, except for the distal surface of the last tooth in each arch.

Class II decay is very common because food and bacteria easily become impacted between the teeth, in the *interproximal* spaces, which are difficult for the patient to clean. (Flossing is the most effective method to remove food particles and debris from interproximal spaces [Figure 8-11].)

Class III (Anterior Teeth Only)

Class III involves the proximal (mesial or distal) surfaces of the anterior teeth (Figure 8-12).

Class IV (Anterior Teeth Only)

Class IV decay involves the interproximal (mesial or distal) surfaces of the anterior teeth *and* the incisal edge or angle. The need for Class IV

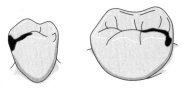

Figure 8-11.   Class II caries on the proximal and occlusal surfaces of bicuspids (premolars) and molars.

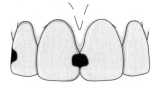

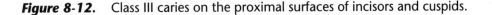

Figure 8-12.   Class III caries on the proximal surfaces of incisors and cuspids.

restorations is often associated with accidental trauma (injury) to the face or mouth (Figure 8-13).

Class V (Anterior and Posterior Teeth)

Class V decay involves the gingival (referring to the gums) one-third of the facial/buccal or lingual surfaces of the teeth. Class V decay most commonly occurs in older adults with gingival recession at the cervical (gingival one-third) portion of the teeth (Figure 8-14).

Class VI

Class VI decay involves the incisal edges or cusp tips of teeth. It is associated with enamel erosion (Figure 8-15).

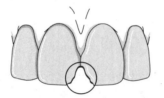

Figure 8-13.   Class IV caries involving the proximal surfaces and incisal edges of central incisors.

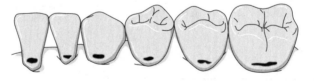

Figure 8-14.   Class V caries involving the gingival or cervical one-third of anterior or posterior teeth.

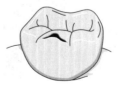

Figure 8-15.   Class VI caries involving defects on incisal edges or cusp tips.

Skill-Building for Success: Student Activities

These optional activities and exercises are designed to help the student put into practice information learned in the chapter.

1. Divide equally numbered groups into class operatories. Wearing personal protective equipment (gloves, masks, and protective eyewear) and using sterilized mouth mirrors, take turns examining each others' mouths. Call out the names of individual teeth as you identify them. Make sure each classmate role plays an "examiner," an "assistant," and a "patient." What did you observe? (If your classroom is not equipped with operatories, you may seat your patients on classroom chairs for examination.)

2. If your program has a human skull, take turns identifying the jaws, the names of the teeth, and the tooth surfaces. If your program does not have a skull, take turns identifying names and surfaces of teeth on a typodont.

Skills Mastery Assessment: Post-Test

Directions: Select the response that *best* answers each of the following questions. Only one response is correct.

1. The office manager must be thoroughly familiar with dental nomenclature to:
   a. interpret the dentist's, hygienist's, or chairside assistant's charting and treatment-related records
   b. provide patients with accurate information in predetermining treatment
   c. bill patients and third-party payors accurately for treatment performed
   d. all of the above

2. The maxilla (jaw bone) is attached to the cranium by a moveable joint called the temporomandibular joint (TMJ).
   a. True
   b. False

3. The maxilla is part of the cranium and is comprised of the hard and soft palate and the maxillary teeth.
   a. True
   b. False

4. All of the following are oral quadrants *except:*
   a. maxillary right
   b. mandibular right
   c. temporomandibular joint
   d. mandibular left

5. Which of the following teeth comprise the anterior sextants?
   a. central incisors
   b. lateral incisors
   c. canines (cuspids)
   d. all of the above

6. The quadrants are determined by an imaginary vertical line dividing the *midline* (front of the face) to designate right and left.
   a. True
   b. False

7. The periodontium consists of all of the following except:
   a. the gingiva
   b. periodontal ligament
   c. the pulp chamber
   d. the alveolar process

8. Which of the following is/are true of enamel? It:
   a. is the hardest substance in the human body
   b. is composed of primarily inorganic materials and is shaped by prismatic rods
   c. protects the tooth
   d. all of the above

9. Which of the following is/are true of dentin? It:
   a. comprises the bulk of the tooth
   b. determines tooth color
   c. registers sensation to pain and temperature
   d. all of the above

10. All of the following are true of cementum *except:*
    a. it is the yellowish-white outer covering of the crown portion of the tooth
    b. it has a porous, rough, textured surface that permits the periodontal fibers to attach
    c. it can rebuild itself, forming secondary cementum
    d. all of the above

11. The dental pulp:
    a. provides the blood and other nutrients from the body to the tooth
    b. is composed of nerve, blood, and lymph
    c. enters the tooth through the apical foramen
    d. all of the above

12. The periodontal ligament acts as a shock absorber to cushion the tooth in the socket and provides attachment to the jawbone.
    a. True
    b. False

13. The area of the pulp that comprises the root(s) is called the pulp chamber.
    a. True
    b. False

14. A cingulum is the lingual lobe of any posterior tooth appearing on the cervical (neck portion) one-third of the tooth.
    a. True
    b. False

15. A developmental groove is a shallow groove or line on the surface of a tooth.
    a. True
    b. False

16. The permanent dentition consists of:
    a. 16 teeth in each arch
    b. eight teeth in each quadrant
    c. 38 teeth in total
    d. a and b only

17. The deciduous or primary dentition consists of:
    a. 10 teeth in each arch
    b. five teeth in each quadrant
    c. a total of 20 teeth
    d. all of the above

18. Commonly referred to as "pit and fissure caries," Class I decay may occur on all of the following *except:*
    a. the occlusal surfaces of bicuspids and molars
    b. the buccal or lingual surfaces of molars
    c. the mesial and/or distal surface of posterior teeth
    d. the lingual surfaces of maxillary incisors

19. Class V decay involves the gingival one-third of the facial/buccal or lingual surfaces of the teeth and is most commonly seen in older adults with gingival recession.
    a. True
    b. False

20. Class III decay involves the incisal edges or cusp tips of teeth and is associated with enamel erosion.
    a. True
    b. False

References

Anderson, P., & Burkard, M. (1995). *The dental assistant* (6th ed.). Albany, NY: Delmar Publishers.

Dietz, E. Tooth morphology: A review of the basics. *The Dental Assistant, The Journal of the American Dental Assistants Association.*

Dofka, C. (1996). *Competency skills for the dental assistant.* Albany, NY: Delmar Publishers.

Chapter 9

Charting the Oral Cavity

- **The Importance of Accurate Clinical Records**
- **The Complete Dental Chart**
- **Tooth Numbering Systems**
  - Universal Numbering System
  - Palmer System
  - Fédération Dentaire Internationale System
- **Charting Symbols and Abbreviations**
  - Anatomic Chart
  - Geometric Chart
- **Office Systems and Color Charting**
- **Charting Terms and Abbreviations**
- **Common Charting Symbols**
  - Caries and Existing Restorations
  - Missing Tooth
  - Tooth to be Extracted
  - Impacted or Unerupted Tooth
  - Drifted Tooth
  - Crown
  - Porcelain-Fused-to-Metal Crown
  - Fixed Bridge
  - Fractured Tooth
  - Periapical Abscess
  - Root Canal
  - Periodontal Pockets
  - Periodontal Abscess

    Overhanging Margin
    Full or Partial Denture
    Implant
- **Manual Charting**
- **Computer-Assisted Charting**
- **Voice-activated Computer-assisted Charting**
    Victor Voice Chart System™
- **Semi-automated Examination Instruments**
    Florida Probe™
    Interprobe™
    Pocket Recording Temperature System
- **American Dental Association (ADA) Coding System**

Learning Objectives

Upon completion of this chapter, the student will achieve an 80 percent or higher score on the Skills Mastery Assessment Post-Test *covering the following material.*

1. Explain the importance of accurate charting records.
2. Describe and differentiate the three most commonly used tooth numbering systems: the Universal System, Palmer System, and Fédération Dentaire Internationale System, and how they are used in charting methods.
3. Be familiar with manual, electronic, and voice-activated charting methods.
4. Demonstrate accurate charting of existing dental restorations, caries, and required treatment using accepted charting symbols, terms, and abbreviations.
5. Demonstrate knowledge in interpreting charted dental information to communicate planned treatment information accurately to other team members and to educate patients about the dentist's recommended treatment plan, as well as treatment completed.

Key Terms

anatomic dental chart	Palmer System
crown	periodontal
extraction	porcelain-fused-to-metal crown
Fédération Dentaire Internationale System	probe systems
	unerupted
fixed bridge	Universal System
geometric dental chart	voice-activated charting
impacted	

The Importance of Accurate Clinical Records

Accurate clinical records are the mainstay of the dental practice. The office manager should be able to review a patient's chart, and then understand, explain, and interpret the patient's necessary (planned) treatment, as well as treatment already completed. Clinical records are generated either manually or electronically, using a system of words, numbers, letters, symbols, or commands that comprise the practice's charting system. Before proceeding with this chapter, the student is advised to work through *Chapter 8, Dental Nomenclature and Related Terminology*.

Thorough understanding of charting includes knowledge of the individual names of the teeth in the primary and secondary dentitions, familiarity with the names of related oral structures and their use and function, knowledge of the names of the surfaces and edges of the teeth, knowledge of the six cavity classifications, and abbreviations of various terms used in preparing and completing patients' records.

Once familiar with this information, the office manager is able to accurately interpret the dentist's planned treatment and to present this information to patients and insurance carriers using both layman's terms and professional terminology appropriately. She or he also uses this information to process manual and electronic claims accurately to third-party carriers (insurance companies). Finally, the office manager must be able to interpret and understand chart notations and accurately describe treatment completed.

The dental chart is a permanent record of the patient's oral condition(s), existing restorations, and diagnosed need for treatment. The dentist's diagnosis is based upon clinical visual examination, review of diagnostic records (including radiographs and study models), the patient's health history, and any symptoms or complaints reported by the patient.

As addressed in *Chapter 2, Legal and Ethical Issues and Responsibilities,* keeping accurate, detailed and up to date clinical records is the first line of defense in reducing the risk of malpractice suits. Neither the office manager nor any other member of the dental team should ever attempt to falsify or alter clinical charting and notations.

If done manually, charting and other clinical notations must be made in ink (note, however, that red ink does not photocopy well). If an error is to be corrected or a change made in the chart notations, a single line should be drawn through the error with the initials of the person entering the notation and the correction made immediately beside it.

Records are the property of the practice and the information contained in them is confidential. Information should not be released except when requested in writing by the patient, another treating dentist, a third-party carrier, or when subpoenaed by an attorney or State Board of Dental Examiners. When forwarding records, the office manager should always send duplicates, never the originals!

The Complete Dental Chart

The complete dental chart provides additional information about the patient, including the area for clinical examination markings that correspond to the teeth. Typically, information included on the clinical chart includes:

- *The patient's personal information* – including name, address, and home and work telephone numbers.
- *Specific medical history* – with notations of importance to the dentist, such as known allergies, current medications prescribed by a physician, blood pressure reading, and the patient's family physician. *Note*: The office manager should update this information at each recall visit, or at least annually.
- *The charting area* – with the actual tooth chart and room for other notations related to clinical findings.
- *Treatment entry area* – indicates dates of service, treatment, or procedure performed, and types of impression, restorative, and anesthetic materials used.

- *The remarks area* – indicating teeth to be watched or other clinical or treatment notations made by the dentist. *Note:* Personal remarks or observations about the patient should *not* be made in this area. If other observations or anecdotal information are to be made, they should be entered on a separate piece of paper and included in the file jacket—never entered into the clinical records. This is to prevent embarrassment to the practice should the records be transferred to another office or should they be subpoenaed.

Tooth Numbering Systems

Charting is based upon tooth numbering systems. Three accepted dental numbering systems are used for dental charting. Most dentists use the system they learned in dental school. While no two dental practices use exactly the same charting methods, following are the most commonly used numbers, symbols, terms, and abbreviations.

It is important for the office manager to remember that dental charting is performed as one faces the patient, that is, left and right are reversed when charting notations are entered. Starting with the last tooth in the *upper right quadrant,* charting entries begin on the *upper left of the dental chart or computer screen.*

Universal Numbering System

The **Universal System** was adopted by the American Dental Association in 1968 as a uniform way for dental practitioners, insurance carriers, and other professionals to communicate using the same language. The intent of the Universal System is to avoid confusion by assigning each tooth in the permanent dentition its own *number,* from #1 to #32. Each tooth in the deciduous dentition has its own *letter,* from A to T.

In the permanent dentition, the teeth are assigned a number starting with the upper right third molar, which is #1. The numbers follow (from #1 through #16) sequentially around the entire maxillary arch to the upper left third molar. Next, the Universal System drops down to the mandibular arch, starting directly below at the lower left mandibular third molar, which is #17. The Universal System continues from the lower left third molar all the way around the mandibular arch to the lower right third molar. The mandibular arch comprises tooth #17 through #32 (Figure 9-1).

MAXILLARY ARCH

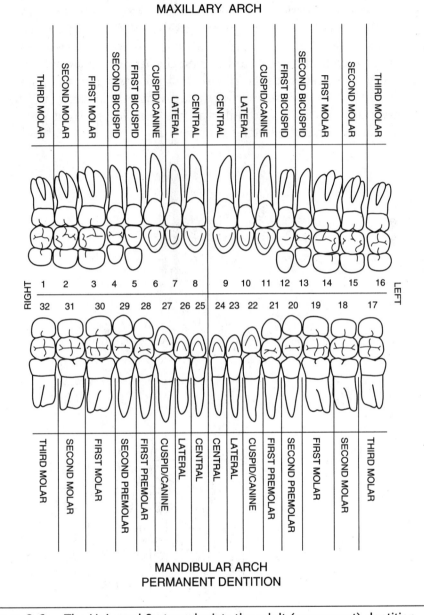

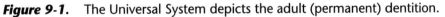

MANDIBULAR ARCH
PERMANENT DENTITION

Figure 9-1. The Universal System depicts the adult (permanent) dentition.

The designations of the Universal System for deciduous or primary teeth follow the same pattern. Starting with the upper right second deciduous molar, the letters begin with *A* and work all the way around the maxillary arch to the upper left second deciduous molar, which is letter *J*. The Universal System drops down to the mandibular arch, starting with the lower left second deciduous molar, which is letter *K*, and follows all the way around the mandibular arch to the lower right second deciduous molar, which is the letter *T* (Figure 9-2).

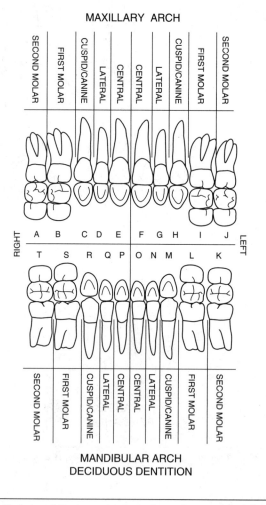

MAXILLARY ARCH

MANDIBULAR ARCH
DECIDUOUS DENTITION

Figure 9-2. The Universal System depicts the primary (deciduous) dentition.

Palmer System

Prior to the acceptance of the Universal System, many dentists used the **Palmer System** of tooth numbering and lettering. Today, many practices still use it. It is especially popular with orthodontists.

In the Palmer System, each tooth in the *quadrant* has a designated number or letter and a *bracket* indicating the quadrant. Starting with the central incisor and working back in each quadrant to the third molar, the teeth in the adult (permanent) dentition are designated from the central incisor as #1 to the third permanent molar #8. A bracket designates the quadrant (Figure 9-3, Table 9-1).

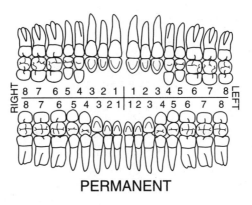

PERMANENT

Figure 9-3.   The Palmer System depicts the adult (permanent) dentition.

Table 9-1   Palmer System

The following table represents tooth numbers by *quadrant,* using the Palmer System.

Adult (Permanent) Dentition:

Central Incisor – #1	Second Bicuspid (second premolar) – #5
Lateral Incisor – #2	First Permanent Molar – #6
Canine (Cuspid) – #3	Second Permanent Molar – #7
First Bicuspid (first premolar) – #4	Third Permanent Molar – #8

Primary (Deciduous) Dentition:

Central Incisor – A	First Deciduous Molar – D
Lateral Incisor – B	Second Deciduous Molar – E
Canine (Cuspid) – C	

In the primary (deciduous) dentition, the Palmer System starts with the central incisor, letter *A* and works back to the second deciduous molar, letter *E,* with a bracket designating the quadrant (Figure 9-4).

Fédération Dentaire Internationale System

The **Fédération Dentaire Internationale System** is a modified version of the Palmer System for the permanent (adult) teeth. Brackets are replaced by quadrant numbers, representing the *first digit* of the numbering system. The quadrants of the permanent mouth are numbered as follows:

Quadrant #1 – maxillary right

Quadrant #2 – maxillary left

Quadrant #3 – mandibular left

Quadrant #4 – mandibular right

The *second digit* is patterned after the Palmer System of tooth #1 through #8, with the central incisor as tooth #1 and the third permanent molar as tooth #8 in each quadrant.

Thus, the first number of each adult tooth ranges from #1 to #4, corresponding to the quadrant; the second number represents the individual tooth number within the quadrant, from #1 to #8.

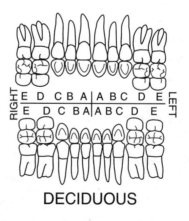

DECIDUOUS

Figure 9-4.   The Palmer System depicts the primary (deciduous) dentition.

The International System starts with the maxillary right central incisor as tooth #11 and follows the quadrant back to the maxillary right third molar, which is #18.

In quadrant #2, the teeth again start at the midline with the maxillary left central incisor as tooth #21 through the maxillary left wisdom tooth, which is #28.

In quadrant #3, the teeth start at the midline with the mandibular left central incisor, which is #31 and goes back to the mandibular left third molar, which is #38.

In quadrant #4, the teeth start at the midline with the central incisor as tooth #41 to the mandibular right third molar, which is tooth #48 (Figure 9-5).

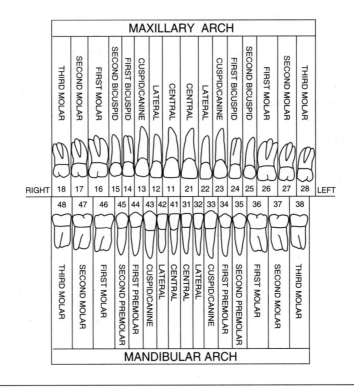

Figure 9-5. The Fédération Dentaire Internationale System depicts the adult (permanent) dentition.

In the Fédération Internationale System, the primary dentition uses quadrant #5 through #8 as follows:

Quadrant #5 – maxillary right
Quadrant #6 – maxillary left
Quadrant #7 – mandibular left
Quadrant #8 – mandibular right

The deciduous teeth are numbered with the quadrant number as the first digit and the tooth number as the second digit, starting with the central incisor in each quadrant as #1 and the second deciduous molar as tooth #5.

The teeth in the maxillary right quadrant start with the first digit #5 (representing the quadrant number) and the second number to indicate the tooth in the quadrant. Thus, the teeth in the maxillary right quadrant comprise #51 through #55, starting with the upper right deciduous central incisor and ending with the maxillary right second deciduous molar, #55.

In the maxillary left quadrant, the teeth begin with the maxillary left deciduous incisor, tooth #61, and end with the maxillary left second deciduous molar, tooth #65.

In the mandibular left quadrant, the teeth start with the mandibular left central incisor, #71, and end with the mandibular left second deciduous molar, tooth #75.

The final quadrant, the mandibular right, is designated by the right central incisor, #81, and ends with the mandibular right second deciduous molar, tooth #85 (Figure 9-6).

Charting Symbols and Abbreviations

Having familiarity with tooth numbering systems, the office manager must next become familiar with charting symbols and other abbreviations used in charting the oral cavity.

There are many different types of dental charts, supplied by a variety of dental forms manufacturers and dental software providers. The two general types of charts are *anatomic* and *geometric*.

Anatomic Chart

The **anatomic dental chart** depicts the teeth and related oral structures as they generally appear upon clinical examination, that is with cusps,

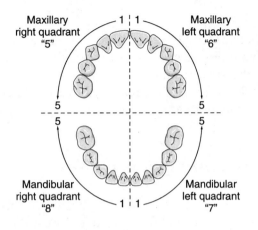

Figure 9-6. The Fédération Dentaire Internationale System depicts the primary (deciduous) dentition.

grooves, pits, and other oral landmarks. Some anatomic charts depict a portion or all of the tooth roots. When charting, the chairside dental assistant fills in the surfaces on the corresponding anatomic areas as directed by the dentist (Figure 9-7).

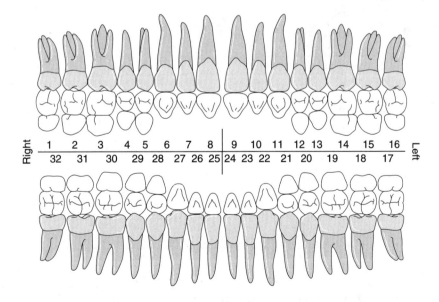

Figure 9-7. A sample anatomic chart.

Geometric Chart

The **geometric** ("circle") **dental chart** depicts each individual tooth as a circle within another circle. Inside this geometric representation are lines that delineate the surfaces and incisal edges of the teeth. When charting, the dental assistant fills in the area inside the circle or lines in the space to correspond to the tooth as directed by the dentist (Figure 9-8).

Office Systems and Color Charting

Although there are many types of charting symbols and ways to indicate specific findings, the office manager must become accustomed to the method the dentist prefers. Many practices use specific colors in the charting area to designate clinical findings. This is to eliminate confusion between treatment required and treatment completed.

Red indicates carious lesions/areas or a tooth requiring treatment. *Blue* indicates existing restorations; direct restorations are colored in, indirect restorations are outlined with cross-hatching. *Green* is sometimes used to depict existing restorations in new patients, and also to depict a *veneer,*

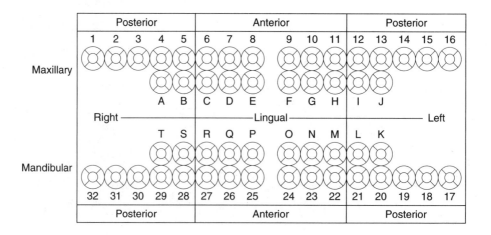

Figure 9-8. A sample geometric chart.

which is outlined, but not colored in. As treatment is completed, the areas charted in red are colored over using blue to indicate the required treatment was completed. The chairside assistant outlines and fills in the areas as dictated by the dentist.

Charting Terms and Abbreviations

It is helpful for all members of the dental team to use a standard set of abbreviations and symbols when charting. This enhances communication and assists the office manager when explaining required treatment to the patient, especially in numbers of surfaces requiring restoration, in developing payment estimates based upon the number of surfaces to be restored, and when filing third-party claims for reimbursement (Table 9-2).

Table 9-2 Common Dental Terms and Abbreviations Used for Charting

Abscess	Abs
Adjustment	Adj
Amalgam	Amal or AM
Anesthetic	Anes
Anterior	Ant
Bitewing	BWX or BW
Bridge	Br
Buccal	B or buc
Cement	Cem
Composite	Com
Consultation	Consult
Crown	Cr or CRN
Deciduous	Decid
Delivery	Del
Denture	Dent
Diagnosis	Diag or DX
Distal	D or Dis
Examination	EX or Exam

Table 9-2 (Continued)

Extraction	Ext or Exo
Estimate	Est
Facial (buccal or labial)	F or Fac
Fluoride	Fl
Fixed bridge	Fix Br
Fracture	FX
Full gold crown	FGCr
Full lower denture	FLD
Full-mouth X-rays	FMX
Full upper denture	FUD
Gold	G
Gold inlay	GI
Gold onlay	GO
Impaction	Impac
Implant	IMPL
Impression	IMP
Incisal	I
Inlay	In
Labial	L or La
Laser	LS
Lidocaine	Lido
Lingual	L or Li
Mesial	M or Mes
Missing	Miss
Nerve block	Nbk
Nitrous oxide	N_2O_2
Occlusal	O or Occ
Onlay	On
Oral home instructions	OHI
Panorex	Pano
Partial lower denture	PLD
Partial upper denture	PUD

Periodontal screening record	PSR
Permanent	Perm
Pit and fissure sealants	PFS
Porcelain	Porc
Porcelain fused to gold	PFG
Porcelain fused to metal	PFM
Porcelain jacket crown	PJC
Posterior	Post
Postoperative	PO
Preparation	Prep
Preventive Oral Hygiene	POH
Prophylaxis	P or PX
Proximal	Prox
Removable	Rem
Root canal therapy	RCT or RC
Seat (final cementation)	St
Shade	Sh
Study models	SM
Temporary	Temp
Tooth	The
Treatment	TX
Treatment Plan	Tx Pl
Xylocaine	Xylo
Zinc-oxide eugenol	ZOE
Zinc oxyphosphate	ZnP

Some abbreviations are used together in describing multiple surfaces of teeth. For example, when compound surfaces of decay are involved, as in a *mesial occlusal distal* restoration, the names of the surfaces are combined and referred to as *mesio-occluso-distal*. (When combining surfaces, the *"al"* is dropped and replaced with an *"o."*) This is abbreviated *"MOD"* with each letter pronounced individually, as *"M"-"O"-"D"* (not *"mod"*). A *distal occlusal* restoration is referred to as *"disto-occlusal"* and is pronounced *"D"-"O"* (not *"do"*).

The most common abbreviations of combined (complex) tooth surfaces are as follows:

- Mesio-occlusal (**MO**) pronounced *"M"-"O"*
- Disto-occlusal (**DO**) pronounced *"D"-"O"*
- Mesio-occluso-distal (**MOD**) pronounced *"M"-"O"-"D"*
- Mesio-incisal (**MI**) pronounced *"M"-"I"*
- Disto-incisal (**DI**) pronounced *"D"-"I"*
- Disto-lingual (**DL**) pronounced *"D"-"L"*
- Bucco-occlusal (**BO**) pronounced *"B"-"O"*
- Linguo-occlusal (**LO**) pronounced *"L"-"O"*

With practice, all members of the dental team quickly learn to use consistent terminology and abbreviations.

Common Charting Symbols

Following are the most commonly used charting symbols. It is important for the dental office manager not only to know how to enter these symbols onto a chart (either manually or electronically) but also to be able to interpret them.

Caries and Existing Restorations

Outline existing decayed surfaces on the chart. Outline and fill in the surfaces filled with amalgam, composite, glass ionomer, or temporary restorations.

Missing Tooth

A missing tooth is one that has been surgically extracted or never formed. Some practices draw an "X" through the full length of the tooth (Figure 9-9); others draw an "X" only through the root area of the tooth.

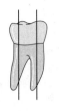

Figure 9-9. A missing tooth.

Figure 9-10. A tooth to be surgically removed (extracted).

Tooth to be Extracted

A tooth scheduled for **extraction** is one that is nonrestorable, infected, or impacted. Draw one or two red diagonal vertical lines through the full length of the tooth (Figure 9-10).

Impacted or Unerupted Tooth

A tooth that is locked into bone is **impacted.** A tooth that has formed but has not appeared in the oral cavity is **unerupted.** Draw a circle around an impacted or unerupted tooth. Include an arrow to indicate the direction of the impaction (Figure 9-11).

Drifted Tooth

A tooth that has moved from its original position in the oral cavity, usually a result of other teeth missing or periodontal disease, is described as having *drifted.* A tooth may drift *downward, upward, forward (mesially),* or *backward (distally).* Indicate the direction of a drifted tooth with an arrow (Figure 9-12).

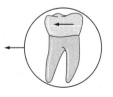

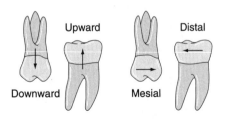

Figure 9-11. A tooth that is either unerupted or impacted.

Figure 9-12. Drifting teeth are indicated with an arrow in the direction of the drift.

Crown

When a tooth has had the clinical portion of the natural enamel reduced and replaced with an artificial covering, that replacement is called a **crown**. A crown that covers three-quarters of a tooth is called a three-quarter crown. A crown that completely covers the clinical crown is a called a full crown. Draw a line around the portion of the natural tooth that has been crowned; cross-hatch marks may be added (Figure 9-13). *Note:* Some practices distinguish porcelain (nonmetallic) crowns with dots drawn through the crown and horizontal lines through gold or metal.

Porcelain-Fused-to-Metal Crown

A crown that is made of porcelain material fused to metal in the laboratory is called a **porcelain-fused-to-metal crown**. Draw a line around the portion of the natural tooth that has been crowned; draw parallel diagonal lines to indicate the portion of metal (Figure 9-14).

Fixed Bridge

A **fixed bridge** contains a minimum of one *abutment tooth* (anchor tooth that is crowned) and one *pontic* (a false tooth that replaces a missing natural tooth). To chart a fixed bridge, draw an X through all the missing natural teeth. Indicate the abutments by outlining them and drawing parallel diagonal lines through the crowned portions. Draw two parallel horizontal lines through all the teeth that comprise the bridge (Figure 9-15).

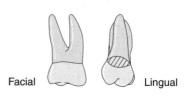

Facial   Lingual

Figure 9-13. A tooth with a crown.   **Figure 9-14.** A porcelain-fused-to-metal crown.

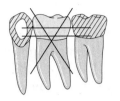

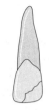

Figure 9-15.   A fixed bridge.

Figure 9-16.   A fractured tooth.

Fractured Tooth

Sometimes teeth become fractured, usually due to physical *trauma* (accident or injury) or sometimes due to advanced decay, biting force, or desiccation (drying out) as a result of root canal therapy. Draw a single jagged line on the chart through the area of the tooth fractured (Figure 9-16).

Periapical Abscess

A periapical abscess forms around the apex (tip) of the root portion of the tooth. On radiograph, it often appears as a darkened round mass. To chart a periapical abscess, draw a small (red) circle around the tip of the abscessed root (Figure 9-17).

Root Canal

A tooth that has received root canal therapy is one that has received *endodontic* treatment. Indicate a root-canal-treated tooth by drawing a single straight vertical line through each root of the tooth. Blue indicates the root canal has been completed; red indicates the root canal is yet to be completed (Figure 9-18).

Figure 9-17.   An apical abscess.

Figure 9-18.   A tooth with root canal therapy.

Periodontal Pockets

A tooth with **periodontal** pockets has some degree of inflammation or stage of infection, commonly referred to as periodontal disease. Periodontal pockets are measured in millimeters. Chart a periodontal pocket by drawing a diagonal line in the pocket area; indicate the number of millimeters next to the line (Figure 9-19).

Periodontal Abscess

A *periodontal abscess* is an infection involving the gingival tissue around the tooth. To chart a periodontal abscess, draw a small (red) circle in the area of the abscess (Figure 9-20).

Overhanging Margin

An overhanging margin on a tooth occurs due to overfilling, thermal expansion of a restorative material, or improper carving of the restoration at the time of placement. To indicate an overhanging margin, draw a small shaded triangle in the area of the overhang (Figure 9-21).

Full or Partial Denture

When natural teeth have been lost, they may be replaced by a removable full or partial denture. Draw a bracket to indicate a full or partial denture (Figure 9-22).

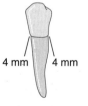

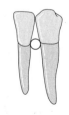

Figure 9-19. A tooth with periodontal pocket(s).

Figure 9-20. A small circle indicates a periodontal abscess.

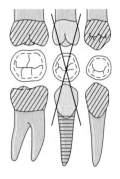

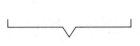

Figure 9-21. Shaded triangles indicate over-hanging margins.

Figure 9-22. Brackets indicate a full or partial denture.

Figure 9-23. Chart an implant by drawing a post where the natural root(s) would appear in bone; chart the remain-der of the tooth as a crown or pontic.

Implant

A dental implant is indicated by drawing a post through the area where the respective tooth root(s) would naturally appear in bone. The area above the surface is charted as a crown (Figure 9-23).

Manual Charting

Traditionally, dental charting was conducted by the dentist's oral dictation of clinical findings to the chairside assistant. The assistant recorded this information onto the clinical record or chart, which was then filed inside a folder or file jacket in a file cabinet in the dental business office. Manual charting is still done in many dental practices today, although the trend is rapidly moving toward full computerization.

Computer-assisted Charting

The computer may be used to store and retrieve collected information dictated by the dentist to the chairside assistant (or dental hygienist) during a patient's oral examination. Once *data* (information) are entered, the computer stores this diagnostic information. Some computers can also compare information collected during successive office visits. One advantage of computer-stored information is that it is faster and more accurate than manual charting. A second advantage is that paperwork is significantly reduced.

Computer *software* (programming entered into the computer's hard drive) can be programmed to compare pre- and postoperative treatment information. This information assists the dentist in planning and initiating treatment. It is also helpful in educating patients about their treatment progress.

The computer can also generate graphic representations, for example, of a patient's periodontal condition. This information may include periodontal pocket depths, gingival bleeding scores, plaque scores, and/or tooth mobility.

Visual graphics are helpful to the dentist and the office manager in providing patient education, explaining treatment plans, and making comparisons of oral health improvement from appointment to appointment. This is also known as a periodontal screening record, or PSR.

Voice-activated Computer-assisted Charting

New advances in technology have made it possible for the dentist to conduct a thorough clinical oral examination and record the information directly into the practice's computer data base for storage and retrieval.

Voice-activated charting is accomplished like manual paper charting, except that all information is input directly into the chairside computer through a microphone headset.

Using specific verbal commands, the operator calls out findings or oral conditions, which are automatically entered into the patient's clinical record in the practice's data base. Specific commands must be learned and used by the operator for this system to work effectively.

Victor Voice Chart System™

The voice-activated computer-assisted vocabulary consists of numbers, anatomical landmarks, and computer commands. It may be used to enter data on pocket depth, tooth mobility, plaque scores, bleeding, missing teeth, restorations, and other related diagnostic information.

Patient education is also available with voice-activated charting using color graphics, information about surgical, endodontic, restorative, periodontal, and implant procedures. One advantage to the practice is time saved by not having to repeat information. Also, the information transfer is paperless.

Some voice-activated systems are programmed by the operator, who speaks directly into a microphone connected to the computer. More sophisticated systems are preprogrammed to recognize a wider speech pattern range, allowing for use by more than one operator in the practice.

While conducting the dental examination, the operator records information by speaking into the microphone. The computer repeats the information, allowing the operator to verify accuracy. If the entry is correct, the operator continues to enter additional information. If the information is incorrect, the operator repeats the entry until it is stored correctly by the computer.

Another advantage to voice-recognition data entry is that the operator can conduct the oral examination and enter data simultaneously. Because the operator does not need to touch pencil, paper, pen, or computer, asepsis is maintained. Patient education is enhanced because the patient hears the information as it is recorded. Use of the voice-activated charting system may also free up the chairside dental assistant's time to perform related duties, such as instrument sterilization, treatment room setup in another operatory, ordering supplies, or processing radiographs.

Semi-automated Examination Instruments

A number of periodontal diagnostic aids further streamline data entry. These instruments record periodontal pocket depth, gingival recession, and attachment loss with a periodontal probe that transmits information directly into the computer.

Probe systems can automatically determine how many millimeters the probe tip is inside the periodontal pocket. The operator manipulates the probe handpiece until it touches a predetermined anatomical landmark on the oral tissue. The computer then calculates the distance from the anatomical landmark to the base of the pocket. The operator presses a foot pedal to record the pocket depth measurement in millimeters. The same land-mark is used at each site during the examination and again at each subse-quent examination. This enables the dentist to compare pocket depth measurements from area to area within the mouth and to record progress and treatment outcomes from appointment to appointment.

An advantage of the semi-automated charting system is it offers accu-racy and repeatability equal to or better than manual probing. The system also generates easy to read charts to assist in patient education.

Florida Probe™

The Florida Probe™ features an autoclavable handpiece that records either *pocket depth* (using the gingival margin as the anatomical landmark) or *gingival attachment level* (using the occlusal surface of the tooth as the anatomical landmark). Because the tips and sleeves of the handpiece are made of titanium, they are compatible with dental implants.

The Florida Probe™ handpiece is connected directly to a laptop or desk-top personal computer terminal in the treatment room and is integratable with both Windows and DOS versions of many other software packages.

The operator uses the system to record the main elements of a peri-odontal examination, including gingival recession, periodontal pocket depth, gingival bleeding, *suppuration* (formation or discharge of pus), tooth mobility, plaque scores, and *furcation* (area where the roots of a mul-tirooted tooth divide) involvement. A multipurpose foot pedal is used to record the information.

The pocket depth and bleeding sites are called out automatically by the computer's voice. The patient hears the clinical findings from the com-puter's voice and visually witnesses the exam on a color monitor. At the completion of the oral examination, the computer generates comprehen-sive graphic and numeric charts of the patient's periodontal condition, identifying the risk stages of periodontal disease.

Interprobe™

The Interprobe™ system employs a disposable probe that automatically records pocket depth and gingival recession. The operator determines the clinical gingival attachment level by combining pocket depth and recession measurements. The Interprobe™'s components are housed in an exam controller unit that fits on most dental bracket tables.

The system uses a lighted panel on the front of the exam controller to direct the operator through the examination. A small screen displays data as it is recorded. Mobility, gingival bleeding, and furcation involvement must then be manually recorded into the exam controller. At the conclusion of the evaluation, computer-generated charts and graphics show the patient's periodontal condition. Changes are recorded from appointment to appointment. The Interprobe™ system can also be connected to a personal computer.

Pocket Recording Temperature System

The PerioTemp™ system records periodontal pocket temperature while a manual probing depth is taken. Pockets with increased levels of periodontal involvement tend to have elevated temperatures. Treatment of periodontal pockets with elevated temperatures reduces the temperature along with other clinical disease indicators, such as inflammation, and subsequently promotes healing.

The PerioTemp™ system allows the dentist to compare the patient's periodontal pocket temperature to the patient's body temperature, thus diagnosing areas of periodontal disease by elevated pocket temperature.

The PerioTemp™ unit has a lighted, color-coded dental chart on the front of its housing, indicating the temperature range of the tooth. *Green* indicates normal; *yellow* indicates slightly above normal; *red* indicates significantly above normal.

A small thermal paper printer is attached to the unit to print out a permanent record of pocket temperatures. This enables the dentist to compare specific pocket temperatures at subsequent visits. The PerioTemp™ features disposable tips that connect to an autoclavable handpiece.

American Dental Association (ADA) Coding System

The American Dental Association publishes a code book (with updates every five years) that lists all known code numbers for dental procedures, by category, specialty, or type of treatment. With repetition, the office manager quickly becomes familiar with the most commonly used ADA codes for procedures. The code system allows third-party payors (insurance companies) to identify procedures by a number, rather than written format. The coding system also saves time when submitting electronic claim forms.

Skill-Building for Success: Student Activities

These optional activities and exercises are designed to help the student put into practice information learned in the chapter.

1. Divide into evenly numbered groups for each operatory available. Wearing appropriate personal protective equipment and using sterilized instruments, take turns role playing the operator, chairside assistant, and patient. The assistant seats and drapes the patient appropriately and passes the mouth mirror and explorer to the operator.

   Using the Universal System, the operator starts at the last tooth in the upper right quadrant. The operator calls out existing restorations by tooth number and surface. The operator also calls out any missing teeth. The chairside assistant records the information onto the patient's chart, using a pencil.

   When the patient's oral charting has been completed, call the instructor over to check the completed charting compared to the patient's mouth. Upon satisfactory completion, the chairside assistant dismisses the patient, removes protective barriers from the equipment, and replaces them with fresh ones. The instrument tray is removed and the contaminated instruments are taken to the instrument sterilization area for processing later.

   Each student takes a turn role playing the operator, patient, and chairside assistant. At the completion of each patient's oral charting exercise, the instructor checks the clinical chart against the patient's oral cavity for accuracy. Any corrections are made. At the completion of the exercise, the dental chart is given to the patient.

2. Your instructor will dictate an oral charting exercise. Complete the charting using the symbols, letters, and abbreviations provided.

Skills Mastery Assessment: Post-Test

Directions: Select the response that *best* answers each of the following questions. Only one response is correct.

1. Clinical records are generated either manually or electronically, using a system of words, numbers, letters, symbols, or commands that comprise the practice's charting system.
   a. True
   b. False

2. Thorough understanding of charting includes:
   a. familiarity with the names of related oral structures and their use and function in the oral cavity
   b. knowledge of the names of the surfaces and edges of all teeth
   c. knowledge of the six cavity classifications
   d. all of the above

3. The office manager must understand charting to do all of the following accurately *except:*
   a. interpret the dentist's planned treatment
   b. present planned treatment information to patients and insurance carriers using both layman's terms and professional terminology
   c. make a proper diagnosis of the patient's oral condition
   d. accurately process manual and electronic claims to third-party carriers

4. The dental chart is a permanent record of:
   a. the patient's oral condition(s)
   b. existing restorations
   c. diagnosed need for treatment
   d. all of the above

5. The dentist's diagnosis is based upon all of the following *except:*
   a. clinical visual examination
   b. the insurance company's recommendations
   c. review of diagnostic records
   d. the patient's health history and any symptoms or complaints reported by the patient

6. When forwarding records, the office manager always sends the originals to ensure accuracy.
   a. True
   b. False

7. Information included on the clinical chart may include:
   a. the patient's personal information and medical history
   b. the charting area
   c. treatment entry area
   d. all of the above

8. Personal remarks about a patient should be entered in the "remarks" area of a clinical chart.
   a. True
   b. False

9. Starting with the last tooth in the upper right quadrant, charting entries begin on the upper left of the dental chart or computer screen.
   a. True
   b. False

10. Using the Universal System, the adult upper right central incisor is tooth:
    a. #1
    b. #16
    c. #8
    d. #11

11. Using the Universal System, the deciduous lower left first molar is tooth letter/number:
    a. K
    b. 74
    c. B
    d. S

12. Using the Palmer System:
    a. each tooth in the *quadrant* has a designated number or letter
    b. each tooth's quadrant is designated by a bracket
    c. each tooth's quadrant is designated by the first digit
    d. a and b only

13. Using the Palmer System, the second bicuspid in *any* quadrant is tooth:

    a. #1

    b. #5

    c. #4

    d. #13

14. In the Fédération Dentaire Internationale System, the mandibular right third molar is tooth:

    a. #16

    b. #8

    c. #48

    d. #58

15. The anatomic dental chart:

    a. depicts the teeth and related oral structures as they generally appear upon clinical examination

    b. depicts the teeth as circular graphics with lines to depict the surfaces and edges of the teeth

    c. provides cusps, grooves, pits, and other oral landmarks, including some or all of the tooth roots

    d. a and c only

16. When marking chart entries, many offices use different colors of pencil or ink to eliminate confusion between treatment required and treatment completed.

    a. True

    b. False

17. As treatment is completed, the areas charted in blue are colored over using red to indicate the required treatment was completed.

    a. True

    b. False

18. The charting abbreviation for full-mouth X-rays is:

    a. BWX

    b. FX

    c. FMX

    d. FUD

19. A missing tooth is indicated on the dental chart by:

    a. drawing a *circle* around the tooth

    b. drawing an X through the tooth

    c. drawing an *arrow* in the space the tooth used to occupy

    d. drawing a *circle* around the tooth and filling in the space with parallel diagonal lines

20. The voice-activated computer-assisted charting vocabulary consists of:

    a. numbers

    b. anatomical landmarks

    c. computer commands

    d. all of the above

References

Anderson, P. C., & Burkard, M. R. (1995). *The dental assistant (6th ed.).* Albany, NY: Delmar Publishers, Inc.

Dofka, C. M. (1996). *Competency skills for the dental assistant.* Albany, NY: Delmar Publishers, Inc.

(1996, June). Early diagnosis of periodontal disease using the Florida Probe system by Computerized Probe, Inc. *Dental Products Report.*

Expanding dental practice with computer technology: Periodontal devices. (1992). Princeton Dental Resource Center.

Ratcliff, P. (1997, October). Early gingival disease: How can we tell the difference? *The Farran Report.*

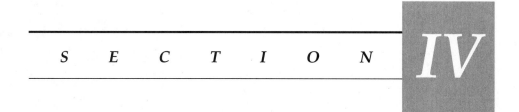

SECTION IV

Business and Financial Records Management

Chapter 10

Patient Records, Diagnosis, and Treatment Planning

- **Filing Systems**
  Filing Safety Rules and Courtesy
  Contents of the Patient File
  Active Files
  Inactive Files
- **Alphabetization**
- **Types of Patient Records**
  Clinical
  Financial Responsibility
  Informed Consent
  Medical/Dental Health History
- **Ownership of Patient Records**
  Transfer of Patient Records
  Retention of Patient Records
- **Diagnosis, Treatment Planning, and Case Presentation**
  Intraoral Dental Radiographs
  Extraoral Radiographs
- **Radiation Safety**
  Protection of the Operator
  Protection of the Patient
  Policy for Protecting Pregnant Patients
- **Radiovisiography: Alternative to Radiographs**
  Digital Radiovisiography Technique
  Prevention of Cross-Contamination with the Digital Radiovisiography
  System

- **Periodontal Disease Predictability Testing**
- **Study Models**
- **Intraoral Camera**
- **The Case Presentation**
- **Recall Program: Lifeline of the Practice**
- **Pharmaceutical Prescriptions**
    Parts of a Pharmaceutical Prescription
    The Office Manager's Responsibility Regarding Prescriptions
- **The Dental Laboratory Prescription**

Learning Objectives

Upon completion of this chapter, the student will achieve an 80 percent or higher score on the Skills Mastery Assessment Post-Test *covering the following material.*

1. Describe types of filing systems and the role of office manager in utilizing and maintaining them.
2. Be familiar with alphabetization and its importance in maintaining patient records.
3. Describe the types of clinical, financial, and medical/dental history forms required in the dental office, and the role of the office manager associated with their use.
4. Describe ownership and confidentiality of patient records and the legal implications.
5. Describe the steps in diagnosis, treatment planning, and case presentation, and the role of the office manager related to them.
6. Be familiar with the most commonly used types of dental radiographs and new technological advances in digital radiography, as well as necessary steps to protect the operator and patient from radiation.
7. Understand the concept of patient referral to a specialist under the direction of the dentist.
8. Describe the office manager's role in maintaining a recall system.
9. List the nine parts of a pharmaceutical prescription and have an understanding of commonly used prescription terms and their meanings.

10. Understand the necessity of a dental laboratory prescription (work order) and the information most commonly required as directed by the dentist. Also, understand the importance of maintaining a lab case tracking system.

Key Terms

case presentation	label
dental radiograph(s)/X-rays	laboratory prescription
diagnosis	pharmaceutical prescription
digital radiography	recall
filing systems	referral
financial history	refill
generic equivalent	signature
heading	study models
health history form	subscription
inscription	superscription
intraoral camera	treatment plan

The role of the dental office manager in setting up and maintaining dental files and patient records is essential. To function smoothly, the well-run dental business office must have sound records management, whether the system is traditional (paper) files or computer-based (paperless).

To ensure the continued smooth running and efficiency of the dental business office, one person in the practice (the office manager) should be responsible for all files and related information. A second dental team member should be cross-trained in records management to ensure continuity in the event of illness or staff turnover.

Filing Systems

Whether the office uses traditional (manual) paper files and filing cabinets or electronically stores and retrieves patient records, the philosophy and format of **filing systems** are similar. Patient files may be *alphabetic,* *numeric,* or *chronological.* Alphabetic is the most common.

If using traditional paper files, the filing system may be either *horizontal* or *vertical.* Stickers are affixed to the side or top of the file folder or jacket, indicating a range of letters beginning the last name, such as *"Ja-Jg"* and *"Jh-Ju."* The labels may also be color coded to assist the office manager in finding a specific patient by range of letters in the last name and the associated color (e.g., *Ja-Jg* may be in red and *"Jh-Ju"* in green). If the office manager were looking for Mr. Jones' file, she or he would rapidly scan the file for a green label with the *"Jh-Ju"* marker.

The office manager will also note that sometimes additional stickers or labels (with or without writing or other identification) may be adhered to the outside of folders to communicate other information understood within the office. These function as a form of silent, color-coded communication that may have meanings such as "penicillin allergy," "public assistance," "difficult patient," "slow pay," "insurance," "prefers nitrous oxide sedation," "patient requires premedication," etc. This system helps ensure patient confidentiality.

Filing Safety Rules and Courtesy

The office manager should follow commonsense safety rules when using a mechanical file. These rules include:

- never leave a file drawer open, as this may cause accidental bruising, tripping, or falling
- never pull out more than one drawer at a time, as this could force the file cabinet to fall over, causing injury
- always return the file promptly to its proper position

It is professional consideration and courtesy never to leave a patient's file out in the open where other people may read the contents. The contents should always be kept confidential.

Contents of the Patient File

The patient file must contain the patient's name (the last name is listed first) and the clinical record, financial responsibility form, informed consent form, medical/dental history form, and necessary **dental radiographs**.

Other personal information, notes, or attributes about the patient should be compiled on a separate piece of paper or on a separate computer document. This may include personal attributes such as hobbies, anecdotal information about patients' personal preferences, family life, or business or civic affiliations. Personal information should *never* be part of the clinical or financial record (Figure 10-1).

Active Files

Active files are those patients of record who have been treated in the office within the past 12 months and/or who owe outstanding fees.

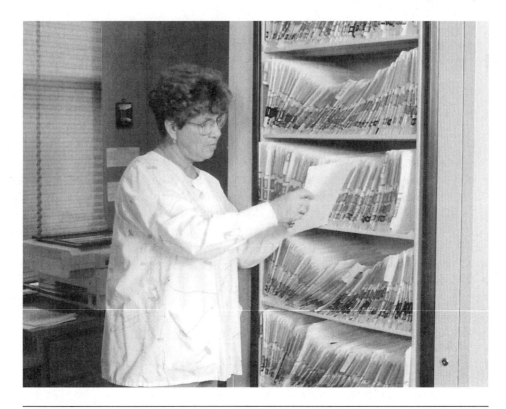

Figure 10-1. The office manager is responsible for maintaining an efficient records management system.

Inactive Files

Inactive files are those patients of record who have not been treated or made contact with the office for more than 12 months prior and have no outstanding balance. Most practices conduct routine computer searches or manual audits of patient files. This is to keep patients from becoming lost in mid-treatment; to see that patients who may have canceled appointments without reappointing are rescheduled to complete treatment; and to ensure that patients are notified of their **recall** appointments when due.

It is the office manager's job to contact and reschedule those patients who have incomplete treatment or who are past due for their recall appointments.

Alphabetization

Knowing proper alphabetization is essential for the office manager to quickly access patient records. Alphabetization is in the following order: the surname (last name), the given name (first name), the middle name or initial, and the patient's title or degree last (Mr., Mrs., Miss, Ms., or Dr.).

The standard rule is "nothing comes before something." As such, "Smith, J." is filed *before* "Smith, John.

When a patient's last name is hyphenated, such as George S. Martin-Jenkins, the hyphenated last name is treated as one name.

When filing the chart of a married woman, her record is filed by her name, not her husband's. Thus, she is "Smith, Charity" and neither "Mrs. Frank T. Smith" nor "Smith, Mrs. Frank T."

If there are two Charity Smiths in the practice, the one with no middle initial is filed first. If there are two Charity Smiths with different middle names, the one with the middle initial or name closer to the beginning of the alphabet is filed first. For example, "Smith, Charity C." is filed before "Smith, Charity S." If two Mrs. Smiths list themselves as "Charity C. Smith" and "Charity Catherine Smith" respectively, the Mrs. Smith with the C. initial is filed ahead of the Mrs. Smith with the full middle name.

Types of Patient Records

While all dental offices are run slightly differently, following are the most commonly used types of dental forms, patient records, and diagnostic aids.

Clinical

Before proceeding, it is recommended the student has reviewed *Chapter 9, Charting the Oral Cavity*. The information covers common components of the clinical record, dental charting, and related terms. The clinical record contains pertinent information resulting from oral examination conducted by the dentist, the patient's report of pain or other complaints (if any), and treatment required or completed.

Each chart entry must be legible, dated, and initialed by the person making the entry.

Financial Responsibility

All patients, whether those of record or new, must complete a financial responsibility form. This information includes the name, address, and phone number(s) of the patient and the responsible party (if different), specific insurance information such as the name of the carrier, the insured's group and/or policy number, and expiration date.

Additional information required includes the responsible party's Social Security number and place of employment. Often a signature is required by the responsible party, agreeing to pay fees not covered by insurance.

The financial responsibility form may also contain specific information about availability of financial payment plans and the office's policy regarding assessment of interest on extended or late payments.

Note that financial records are *not* a part of the clinical record (Figure 10-2).

For additional information on insurance coverage and completing financial forms, refer to *Chapter 12, Managing Accounts Receivable.*

Informed Consent

Prior to initiating treatment, the dentist should also have a signed informed consent form as part of the patient's complete record. Informed consent is addressed in *Chapter 2, Legal and Ethical Issues and Responsibilities.*

Medical/Dental Health History

Prior to examining a patient or initiating treatment, it is essential to have the patient, parent, or legal guardian complete or update a medical/dental

Welcome

We are pleased to welcome you to our practice. Please take a few minutes to fill out this form as completely as you can. If you have questions we'll be glad to help you. We look forward to working with you in maintaining your dental health.

Patient Information

Name _____ Soc. Sec. # _____
        Last Name   First Name   Initial

Address _____

City _____ State _____ Zip _____ Phone _____

Sex ☐ M ☐ F Age _____ Birthdate _____ ☐ Single ☐ Married ☐ Widowed ☐ Separated ☐ Divorced

Patient Employed by _____ Occupation _____

Business Address _____ Business Phone _____

Whom may we thank for referring you? _____

Notify in case of emergency _____ Home Phone _____ Work Phone _____

Primary Insurance

Person Responsible for Account _____
        Last Name   First Name   Initial

Relation to Patient _____ Birthdate _____ Soc. Sec. # _____

Address (if different from patient) _____ Home Phone _____

City _____ State _____ Zip _____

Person Responsible Employed by _____ Occupation _____

Business Address _____ Business Phone _____

Insurance Company _____ Phone _____

Contract # _____ Group # _____ Subscriber # _____

Name of other dependents under this plan _____

Additional Insurance

Is patient covered by additional insurance? ☐ Yes ☐ No

Subscriber Name _____ Relation to Patient _____ Birthdate _____

Address (if different from patient) _____ Soc. Sec. # _____

City _____ State _____ Zip _____ Phone _____

Subscriber Employed by _____ Business Phone _____

Insurance Company _____ Phone _____

Contract # _____ Group # _____ Subscriber # _____

Name of other dependents under this plan _____

Please complete both sides.

Figure 10-2. Sample patient financial responsibility form. *(reprinted courtesy ©SmartPractice, Inc. Phoenix, AZ. All rights reserved. To order call 800-522-0800.)*

health history form. This is to alert the dentist to prescribed drugs currently being taken by the patient, the name and telephone number of the patient's family physician, recent hospitalizations or surgeries, current medical conditions (such as a history of cardiac disease, diabetes, hypertension, hepatitis, or HIV-disease), and any known allergies. The health history form should also contain the name and telephone number of a responsible party to contact in case of an emergency.

The medical/dental history form provides an excellent opportunity to note the patient's feelings and attitudes about his or her teeth, to list current dental complaints, and to record goals for improved oral health.

When necessary, the office manager should assist the new patient in completing this and all other forms and no blank spaces should be left on the form (Figure 10-3).

Note: With the recent rise in latex sensitivity reported by health care workers and *anaphylaxis* reported by patients, it is important to question patients about any known sensitivity to latex products.

Ownership of Patient Records

The *Right to Privacy Act* grants patients access to their personal records, including medical and dental charts. The question occasionally arises, "Who owns the records?" While the patient has the right to review records or to obtain copies of them, the practice owns the records.

Transfer of Patient Records

When a patient changes dentists or relocates, he or she may request the records be transferred to the new treating dentist. The new dentist may request copies of the records. The office manager should request the patient or new dentist to send a written, signed, and dated request for transfer of records. The records may be released either to the new dentist or to the patient. Further, the office manager should send legible, quality duplicates of the records—never the originals! Many practices charge a fee for duplication and mailing costs.

A request for records also occurs when the dentist determines the need for **referral** to another dentist, most often a dental specialist, for further treatment. For additional information about transfer of records, see *Chapter 2, Legal and Ethical Issues and Responsibilities.*

HEALTH HISTORY & REGISTRATION

Patient Number _____ A B C

PATIENT INFORMATION

PATIENT'S NAME Last _____ First _____ Middle Initial _____ SEX: M F BIRTHDATE _____ AGE _____

Soc. Sec. # _____ If Patient is a Minor, give Parent's or Guardian's Name _____ TODAY'S DATE _____

Who May We Thank for Referring You to our Office? _____ Reason for this Visit _____

RESPONSIBLE PARTY INFORMATION

NAME Last _____ First _____ Middle _____ MARITAL STATUS _____

RESIDENCE Street _____ Apt. # _____ City _____ State _____ Zip _____

MAILING ADDRESS Street _____ Apt. # _____ City _____ State _____ Zip _____

HOW LONG AT THIS ADDRESS _____ HOME PHONE _____ WORK PHONE _____

PREVIOUS ADDRESS (if less than 3 yrs.) Street _____ City _____ State _____ Zip _____ How Long _____

SOCIAL SECURITY # _____ BIRTHDATE _____ DRIVER'S LICENSE # _____ RELATION TO PATIENT _____

EMPLOYER _____ OCCUPATION _____ NO. YEARS EMPLOYED _____

RESPONSIBLE PARTY'S SPOUSE

NAME _____ LAST _____ FIRST _____ MIDDLE

EMPLOYER _____ NO. YEARS EMPLOYED _____

OCCUPATION _____ SOC. SEC. # _____

WORK PHONE _____ BIRTHDATE _____

EMERGENCY INFORMATION: RELATIVE NOT LIVING WITH YOU.

| | RELATIONSHIP |

NAME _____

ADDRESS _____

CITY, STATE _____ PHONE _____

DENTAL INSURANCE INFORMATION (Primary Carrier)

Insured's Name _____

Insurance Co. _____

Insurance Co. Address _____

Insured's Employer _____

Insured's Soc. Sec. # _____ Group # _____ Local # _____

If you have double dental insurance coverage, complete this for the second coverage.

Insured's Name _____

Insurance Co. _____

Insurance Co. Address _____

Insured's Employer _____

Insured's Soc. Sec. # _____ Group # _____ Local # _____

It is important that I know about your Medical and Dental History. These facts have a direct bearing on your Dental Health. This information is strictly confidential and will not be released to anyone. Thank you for taking the time to completely fill out this questionnaire.

DENTAL HISTORY	YES	NO
HOW LONG SINCE you have seen a Dentist?		
Last COMPLETE Dental Exam, Date:		
Last FULL MOUTH X-RAYS, DATE: (16 small Films or Panoramic)		
Are you having PROBLEMS now?	☐	☐
WHAT?		
Is your present dental health POOR?	☐	☐
Do you wear DENTURES? (Partials or Full)	☐	☐
Are you UNHAPPY with your dentures?	☐	☐
Would you like to know more about PERMANENT REPLACEMENTS?	☐	☐
Are you APPREHENSIVE about dental treatment?	☐	☐
Have you had any PERIODONTAL (GUM) treatments?	☐	☐
Do your gums BLEED, or feel TENDER or IRRITATED?	☐	☐
Are your teeth SENSITIVE to hot, cold, sweets, pressure? (circle)	☐	☐
Are you UNHAPPY with the APPEARANCE of your teeth?	☐	☐
Are you aware of GRINDING or CLENCHING your teeth?	☐	☐
Do you have HEADACHES, EARACHES, or NECK PAINS?	☐	☐
Have you worn BRACES on your teeth? (ORTHODONTICS)	☐	☐
Do you have DISCOLORED teeth that bother you?	☐	☐
Would you like your smile to LOOK BETTER or DIFFERENT?	☐	☐
Do you REGULARLY use DENTAL FLOSS?	☐	☐

Name of Previous Dentist: _____

City: _____ State: _____

How do you feel about your teeth? _____

Please RANK the following in the order in which they would KEEP YOU FROM having dental treatment.

FEAR of pain	#	LACK of concern	#
COST of treatment	#	MISSING work time	#

MEDICAL HISTORY	YES	NO
Do you have any CURRENT HEALTH PROBLEMS?	☐	☐
Are you under a PHYSICIAN'S CARE now?	☐	☐
For What?		
What MEDICATIONS are you currently taking?		
Are you PREGNANT?	☐	☐
Do you use cigars/cigarettes, pipe or chewing tobacco? Circle	☐	☐

CIRCLE ANY OF THE FOLLOWING WHICH YOU HAVE HAD, OR PRESENTLY HAVE:

Heart Disease or Attack	A.I.D.S./A.R.C./HIV Pos.	Bruise Easily
Angina Pectoris	Hepatitis A (infectious)	Emphysema
High Blood Pressure	Hepatitis B (serum)	Tuberculosis (TB)
Heart Murmur	Liver Disease	Asthma
Rheumatic Fever	Blood Transfusion	Hay Fever
Congenital Heart Lesions	Drug Addiction	Sinus Trouble
Mitral Valve Prolapse	Hemophilia (Bleeding Problems)	Allergies or Hives
Artificial Heart Valve	Fever Blisters	Thyroid Disease
Heart Pacemaker	Epilepsy or Seizures	Radiation Treatment
Heart Surgery	Nervousness	Arthritis
Artificial Joints (Hip, Knee)	Psychiatric Treatment	Cortisone Medicine
Anemia	Glaucoma	Pain in Jaw Joints
Stroke	Chemotherapy (Cancer, Leukemia)	Alcoholism
Kidney Trouble	Venereal Disease	Cosmetic Surgery
Ulcers	(Syphilis, Gonorrhea, etc.)	

ARE YOU ALLERGIC TO OR HAVE YOU REACTED ADVERSELY TO ANY OF THE FOLLOWING MEDICATIONS?

Aspirin	Local Anesthetic	Erythromycin
Nitrous Oxide	Codeine	Penicillin

Are you aware of being allergic to any other medications or substances?

If yes, please list: _____

Is there any other Medical or Dental information that you feel I should know about?

FAMILY PHYSICIAN _____ PHONE NO. _____

PATIENT Signature (Parent of Child) _____ Date: _____ DENTIST Signature _____

1995© R L C (303) 751-3321

Figure 10-3. Sample medical/dental history form. *(reprinted courtesy ©Smart-Practice, Inc. Phoenix, AZ. All rights reserved. To order call 800-522-0800.)*

Retention of Patient Records

At one time it was thought sufficient to retain patient records for seven years past the last date of treatment. Today it is considered important to retain patient records for 30 years past the last date of treatment or within the statutes of limitation of a specific state (if different).

If the dentist retires, sells, or transfers the ownership of the practice or the dentist passes away, the records become property of the new practice owner.

Diagnosis, Treatment Planning, and Case Presentation

Before the dentist can form a **treatment plan**, he or she must use additional clinical aids to determine a **diagnosis.** These most often include dental radiographs (X-rays) or **digital radiography**, and may also include genetic susceptibility to periodontal disease testing, **study models** (stone or plaster casts of the patient's teeth and supporting structures), and **intraoral camera** images, photos, or video tapes.

Intraoral Dental Radiographs

Dental radiographs are a vital aid for the dentist in making a diagnosis. Because radiographs reveal structures inside the teeth and below the gingiva, they aid in the detection of significant pathology (disease) and other conditions not always apparent upon clinical examination alone.

The most common types of individual dental radiographs (X-rays) used for diagnosis are cavity-detecting *bitewings* (so called because the patient bites down on the side of a film packet tab) and *periapical* (meaning around the tips of the tooth root/s) individual films.

The American Dental Association recommends a *full-mouth series* (or full-mouth survey) for *dentulous* (having natural teeth) adult dental patients every two years or as deemed necessary by the dentist. A full-mouth series of dental X-rays traditionally comprises 14 periapicals (three each maxillary and mandibular anterior films, four each maxillary and mandibular posterior films) and four bitewings (one each of the bicuspids and molars on both left and right sides).

Note that many dentists now include seven bitewings as part of a full-mouth series. (The three additional films comprise anterior bitewings recording the maxillary central incisors, lateral incisors, and cuspids, respectively.)

Bitewing films record the clinical crowns and interproximal areas of teeth. They are used primarily for detection of carious lesions (decay) not visible to the naked eye.

Periapical films are used to examine the entire tooth, including the crown, the root structure, and the supporting structures around the teeth. They are used primarily for diagnosis of periodontal disease and assessment of pathological conditions associated with the loss of supportive bone structure, subgingival and interproximal calculus, changes in pulpal health, and abscesses. They also reveal the effect on the occlusion caused by premature loss or the prolonged retention of deciduous teeth and the consequences of losing the succedaneous teeth (Figure 10-4).

Extraoral Radiographs

Films used to survey the entire oral cavity on one large film placed in a cassette outside the mouth *(extraorally)* are referred to as *panoramic* films. While producing a somewhat enlarged image, panoramic films are *not* as

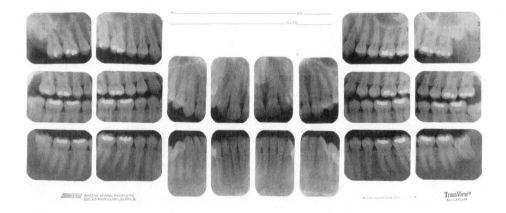
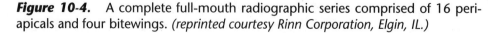

Figure 10-4. A complete full-mouth radiographic series comprised of 16 periapicals and four bitewings. *(reprinted courtesy Rinn Corporation, Elgin, IL.)*

diagnostically accurate as a full-mouth series of individual films. The panoramic film is helpful to the dentist in detecting temporomandibular joint disorders, impactions, orthodontic conditions, supernumerary and unerupted teeth, and pathological (disease) conditions.

On the direction of the dentist, a panoramic film is most often used in conjunction with a minimum of one set of posterior bitewing films (Figure 10-5).

Other types of dental films include *cephalometric* and *occlusal* radiographs.

Radiation Safety

Radiation safety is of primary importance in protecting both dental team members and their patients. Because radiation is *cumulative,* that is, it builds up over time, repeated exposure may eventually cause harmful side effects such as birth defects, skin and eye damage, sterility, hormonal imbalances, blood changes, or cancer in susceptible individuals.

Protection of the Operator

Following are steps the operator or dental assistant radiographer should take to protect himself or herself from the cumulative effects of radiation.

1. Never attempt to hold a film in a patient's mouth during radiographic exposure.
2. Never stand in the direct path of the X-ray beam during exposure.
3. Always stand at a right angle to the X-ray tubehead and a minimum of six to eight feet away from the patient or behind a lead-lined wall or lead shield during exposure. The minimum thickness of the lead lining required in most states is 1/32 of an inch.
4. Ensure the X-ray machine is monitored by an independent examiner according to local or state laws, usually annually.
5. Always wear a monitoring *dosimeter badge* on uniforms or scrubs and send it to an outside monitoring agency for assessment. This badge is monitored monthly and the resulting report provides legal documentation of radiation safety standards in the office (Figure 10-6).

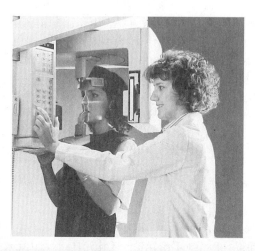

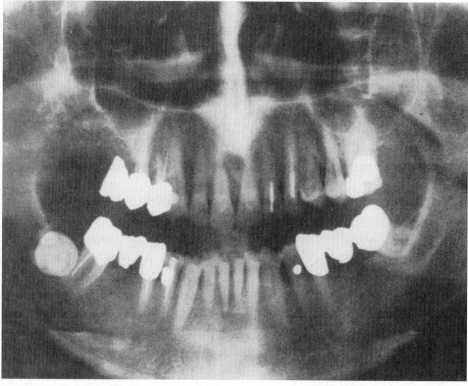

Figure 10-5. A dental assistant exposing an extraoral panoramic radiograph and the resulting film. *(courtesy DENTSPLY International Inc., GENDEX Corporation, Midwest Dental Products Corporation.)*

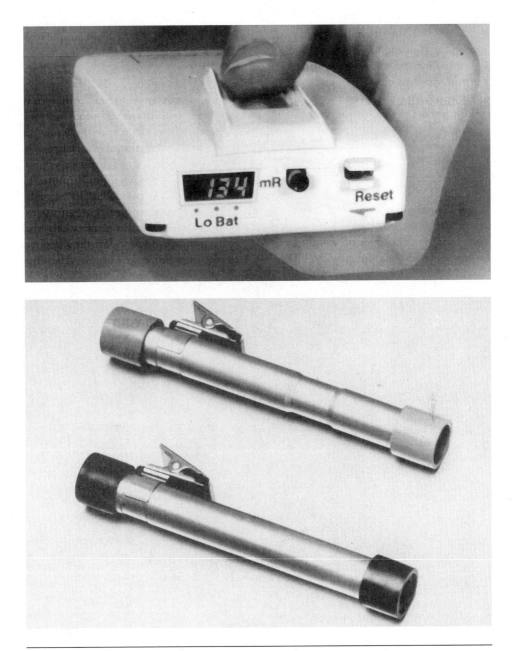

Figure 10-6. Dosimeter badges designated to clip onto the uniform or scrub suit pocket and monitor. The dosimeter records the amount of radiation received during the use period (usually one month). *(Courtesy Nuclear Associates, Carle Place, NY).*

Protection of the Patient

Following are steps the operator or dental assistant radiographer may take to protect patients from radiation.

1. Place a protective lead apron with *thoracic* (pertaining to the throat and upper chest) collar high enough to protect the thyroid gland on all patients being exposed to radiation (Figure 10-7).

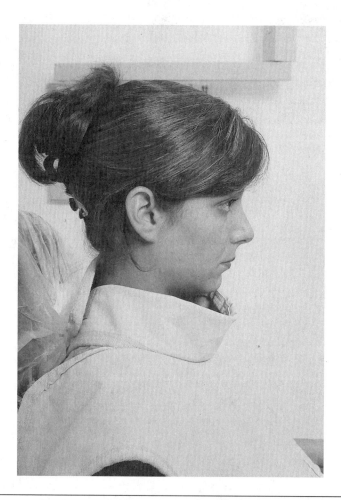

Figure 10-7. A lead apron with thoracic collar protects the patient from additional radiation.

When not in use, store the lead apron over a dowel or on a wooden hanger to prevent cracking of the apron. *Note:* Never fold the lead apron or place it over a hook, as this may result in cracking, puncturing, or tearing of the apron.

2. Take only the minimum number of films required by the dentist.
3. Use proper film positioning, exposure, and processing procedures to reduce the number of retakes.
4. Use the fastest speed film available with the least amount of radiation exposure.

Policy for Protecting Pregnant Patients

Another important aspect of exposing the patient to radiation is the possibility of pregnancy and the increased risk to the unborn child. Thus, it is essential that the office manager take or update each patient's medical history at each recall visit. Many practices display a sign or print a notice on the health history form that indicates *"If you are pregnant or think you may be pregnant, please notify the doctor or a staff member."*

Before exposing radiographs on an expectant patient, the office manager or chairside assistant should alert the dentist, who may wish to consult the patient's obstetrician first. Only if X-rays are absolutely necessary should they be taken on a pregnant patient and then preferably during the second or third *trimester* (three-month duration of pregnancy), when the developing fetus is less susceptible to the effects of radiation.

Radiovisiography: Alternative to Radiographs

Alternative technology called *radiovisiography* (RVG) or *direct digital radiography* (DDR) takes dental X-rays in half the time of traditional films.

The filmless digital system employs a reusable intraoral *sensor* that produces digital radiographic images on a computer monitor. The chairside assistant can use the sensor in conjunction with a traditional X-ray tubehead or with the digital system, which permits automatic activation of the sensor. Digital radiography reduces radiation exposure by 90 percent compared to standard X-ray techniques and also minimizes cross-contamination by eliminating the handling of contaminated film packets (Figure 10-8).

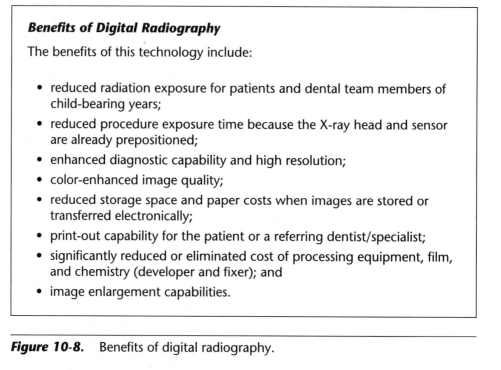

Benefits of Digital Radiography

The benefits of this technology include:

- reduced radiation exposure for patients and dental team members of child-bearing years;
- reduced procedure exposure time because the X-ray head and sensor are already prepositioned;
- enhanced diagnostic capability and high resolution;
- color-enhanced image quality;
- reduced storage space and paper costs when images are stored or transferred electronically;
- print-out capability for the patient or a referring dentist/specialist;
- significantly reduced or eliminated cost of processing equipment, film, and chemistry (developer and fixer); and
- image enlargement capabilities.

Figure 10-8. Benefits of digital radiography.

Digital Radiovisiography Technique

The chairside assistant plugs the sensor directly into the computer and places it in the oral cavity using an *adaptor.* Within a few seconds, the X-ray machine activates and the oral image appears on the computer monitor. A full-mouth series of radiographs can be completed in about half the time required using conventional methods. The images are stored on the computer's hard drive and/or on a tape backup, eliminating the necessity of traditional "paper" files.

Using the paralleling technique, the dental assistant creates *parallelism* between the *long axes* of the teeth and the *sensor,* then directs the X-ray beam at a 90-degree angle to both the teeth and the sensor.

To expose *periapical* films, the chairside assistant mounts the sensor in a *positioner* covered with a disposable clear plastic sheath. She or he then positions the tubehead by resting the cone in the "half-moon" guide attached to the positioner. Within a few seconds after activating the timer switch, the image appears on the monitor screen.

To expose *bitewings*, the assistant uses the computer *mouse* to click once on the icon to select the bitewing format on the upper tool bar. The sensor is sheathed and the flaps are attached to the center of the active side of the sensor. The sensor is placed horizontally between the molars and the patient is instructed to bite down tightly on the foam tabs.

For most adult patients, two bitewings on each side of the mouth are recommended. Only one on each side is recommended for children. The X-ray head is positioned the same as when taking traditional bitewings. The bitewing image appears on the screen within a few seconds of activating the *timer switch.*

Prevention of Cross-Contamination with the Digital Radiovisiography System

To prevent cross-contamination, the dental assistant places a disposable sheath-barrier on the sensor while used in the mouth. At the end of the procedure, the assistant removes the sheath and surface disinfects the sensor after every patient. At the end of the day, the sensor is placed in cold sterilization.

Periodontal Disease Predictability Testing

Periodontal disease predictability testing uses a finger-stick blood test to determine future genetic susceptibility to periodontal disease. The test is used to identify an excess amount of the disease-causing chemical that regulates the body's inflammatory response to bacteria. (Periodontal disease is a reaction between the host and an infection associated with bacteria in dental plaque.)

Early diagnosis of periodontal disease assists the dentist in identifying *at-risk* patients. It is also used as an additional tool for treating patients diagnosed with varying stages of periodontal disease.

A sample of blood is taken from the patient's finger and sent to a laboratory. The test identifies patients who, when infected with bacteria associated with developing periodontal disease, are at risk. The results of periodontal disease predictability testing can be used by the dentist as a form of verification to patients during treatment presentation for the need for further treatment. Patients who are periodontally healthy, with a family history of severe periodontitis, should also be considered candidates for predictability testing.

Regardless of whether patients test positive or negative for periodontal disease predictability, the chairside assistant can provide invaluable instruction and home care education in helping all patients maintain and improve their oral health.

Study Models

Study models are duplicate stone or gypsum models of the patient's teeth and surrounding oral structures. Study models are most often used by orthodontists prior to treatment or by general dentists or prosthodontists for crowns and bridges, full or partial dentures, or implants (Figure 10-9).

Intraoral Camera

The intraoral camera represents a significant breakthrough in diagnosis and treatment plan acceptance. Using a *wand* which is actually a microscopic television camera attached to a *computer* and high-resolution *color monitor*, the operator freezes enlarged dental images (magnified up to 10 times original size) onto the *screen*. The video system uses either a flashing *strobe light* or a *fiber optic light*. These images may be printed out instantly as color photographs, saved in the computer database, or videotaped.

Patient acceptance of recommended treatment increases when patients view individual teeth or a group of teeth and see conditions such as:

- damaged or broken restorations
- gingival inflammation
- various stages of periodontal disease
- outdated or discolored restorations
- dental bone loss
- calculus buildup
- tooth stains and discolorations

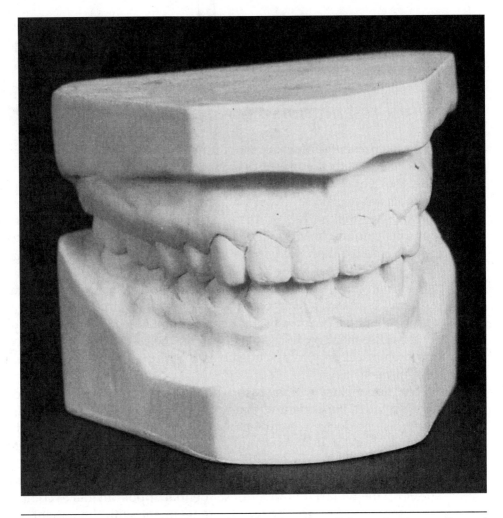

Figure 10-9. Study models are a functional replica of the patient's mouth used in diagnosis, treatment planning, and fabrication of dental prostheses and orthodontic appliances.

- hairline fractures and tooth cracks
- extensive decay
- orthodontic conditions
- missing or drifted teeth
- other oral diseases and conditions

Because use of the intraoral camera to record diagnostic photos and images is not an irreversible procedure, the chairside dental assistant may take and record these images to assist the dentist in making a diagnosis.

The Case Presentation

The **case presentation** is an appointment in which no clinical treatment is performed. With the use of diagnostic aids and charted clinical information, the dentist meets with the patient (and often an accompanying family member) to explain an extensive case. It is the office manager's responsibility to see that all related materials, including the patient's chart, radiographs (mounted on a viewbox), study models, intraoral photos and other demonstration models, patient education brochures, or visual aids, are assembled prior to the appointment.

In many large offices the office manager meets with the patient to explain the doctor's diagnosis and recommended treatment plan. At this appointment the proposed treatment, often planned in phases, is explained by the office manager to the patient. After the case is presented, the patient has the opportunity to ask questions regarding treatment, fees, and time commitment.

At the conclusion of the case presentation appointment, the office manager provides the patient with a written treatment plan estimate. In some practices, the doctor recommends alternate treatment plans, providing the *preferred* form of treatment and *alternative* treatments. The patient then makes a decision, often based upon financial resources.

It is the office manager's job to ensure that a treatment plan is accepted, to set up the required number of sequential appointments to complete the treatment, and to make financial arrangements with the patient. *Note:* To prevent misunderstandings, complete financial arrangements must be made by the office manager and communicated verbally and in writing prior to commencing with treatment. For additional information on financial arrangements, see *Chapter 12, Managing Accounts Receivable.*

Recall Program: Lifeline of the Practice

Recalls are addressed in a number of areas throughout this text. *Recall program* means once a patient has completed current necessary treatment, he or she will be "recalled" to the practice in the future for the next oral examination, prophylaxis, or subsequently required radiographs or treatment. Some practices use the term "recare" appointment.

In most practices, recall duration is six months. For some patients with periodontal conditions, this period may be every three or four months. The office manager is responsible for maintaining patient records and notifying patients of their recall appointments.

Whether the system is managed manually or by computer, the two most common methods of recalling patients are by *prebooking* the next due recall (the subsequent number of months ahead) or by notifying the patient when the next recall appointment is due, either by telephone or mail. If recalls are handled manually, most office managers use a system where the patient's notice is filed six months from the date of completed treatment. For example, if the patient's restorative treatment is completed in May and he or she is due to be recalled in six months, the office manager files the recall notice behind the November tab of the recall file tab (Figure 10-10).

If the practice uses a computer system to print out recall notices and/or labels, the office manager inputs the information by month due and prints out the list by month when the notice is due. She or he then either mails out recall notices (usually postcards) or telephones the patient to schedule the recall appointment.

Pharmaceutical Prescriptions

The office manager must also understand the importance of the information required when the dentist writes a prescription for a *controlled* drug. (A controlled drug is one that requires the prescription of a licensed doctor; the drug is not available over the counter in a pharmacy.)

Before writing any prescription, the doctor should double-check the patient's health history for drug interactions, reactions, or allergies reported.

Note: It is illegal for anyone other than the dentist (who has a narcotics license) to write (sign), phone in to a pharmacy, or dispense *any* controlled drugs for a patient. Any deviation from this may result in the dentist's loss of prescription-writing privileges or other restriction of practice.

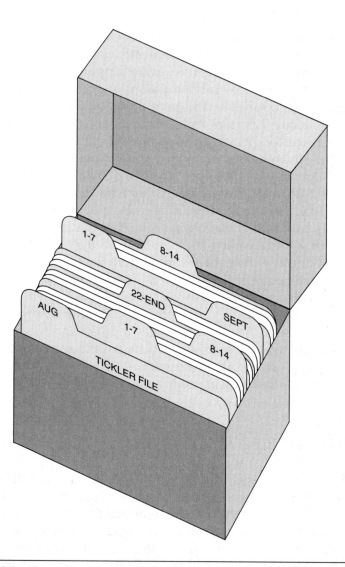

Figure 10-10. Sample manual "R.S.V.P." recall file index system. *(reprinted courtesy ©SmartPractice, Inc. Phoenix, AZ. All rights reserved. To order call 800-522-0800.)*

In dentistry, drugs are most often prescribed for *pain control* and *infection.* Occasionally, they may be prescribed for *anxiety* reduction in patients requiring mild sedation. Premedication with prophylactic antibiotics of patients with certain joint replacements, heart valve replacements, and other cardiac conditions such as a history of rheumatic fever, must also be noted on the patient's chart. Antibiotics must be prescribed and taken by the patient approximately one hour prior to the appointment. It is the office manager's responsibility to alert both the patient and the dentist when contacting the patient to confirm the appointment 24 hours in advance. This is to ensure that the patient picks up the prescription from the pharmacy and takes the medication one hour prior to the appointment.

Parts of a Pharmaceutical Prescription

A **pharmaceutical prescription** has nine parts. The office manager must be familiar with them and be able to interpret their contents and meaning, especially if patients ask questions regarding their prescriptions.

1. The **heading** – contains the doctor's name, degree (DDS or DMD), office address, and telephone number.

2. The **superscription** – includes the date of the prescription, the patient's name, address, age, and gender.

3. The **inscription** – the portion of the prescription that contains the name of the drug, dosage form, and the amount of the dose. Abbreviations are usually used when writing the inscription, such as *"Penicillin V 250 mg tabs"* (Figure 10-11).

4. The **subscription** – the portion of the prescription that contains the amount of the drug and directions for preparation of the drug for dispensing. The subscription may include *"dispense #30."* The number indicates the number of tablets or capsules to be dispensed in the bottle. If the prescription is for a liquid, the volume to be dispensed is indicated in this area.

5. The **signature** – is derived from the Latin word *Signum* and is abbreviated *Sig* or *S*; it is followed by specific directions about how the drug is to be taken. The word signature directs what is to be printed on the pharmacy label affixed to the container. An example of a signature is: *"Sig: tabs 1 q4h,"* which means: *"take one tablet every four hours."*

6. The **label** – the part of the prescription that describes the contents. An example of the information is: *"Ibuprofen 800 mg."* The label may also contain the dose, for example, 250 mg or 500 mg.

Common Prescription Abbreviations

Abbreviation	Meaning
ac	before meals
bid	twice a day
caps	capsules
liq	liquid
ml	milliliter
pc	after meals
q2h	every two hours
q3h	every three hours
q4h	every four hours
q6h	every six hours
q12h	every 12 hours
qd	daily
qh	every hour
qid	four times a day
prn	as necessary, when necessary
stat	immediately
tabs	tablets
tid	three times a day
tsp	teaspoon

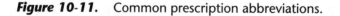

Figure 10-11. Common prescription abbreviations.

7. The **refill** – the part of the prescription where the dentist indicates the number of refills (if any) to be dispensed.

8. The designation for filling the prescription with a **generic equivalent** drug – the portion of the prescription in which the dentist indicates whether the pharmacist must dispense the prescription as written (when a trade name or brand name is used) or if a generic equivalent may be substituted. Note, not all brand name drugs have generic equivalents. A generic equivalent drug is non-brand name protected and is less expensive.

9. The doctor's actual signature and *DEA number*. The dentist must have a current DEA (Drug Enforcement Agency) license to write prescriptions.

The Office Manager's Responsibility Regarding Prescriptions

The office manager must ensure that all information relating to prescription drugs written by the dentist is recorded properly in the patient's chart. This is for legal documentation, to avoid confusion later on, and also to prevent any misunderstandings or reduce the likelihood of subsequent drug interactions or overdoses.

Many offices use a *duplicate prescription pad system* in which the top portion is given to the patient and the bottom copy is placed in the patient's permanent file jacket. Numbering of prescriptions is also routinely done by many offices as a tracking system to monitor writing of prescriptions and to reduce the likelihood of stolen or forged prescriptions.

The office manager should take steps to ensure that the dentist's prescription pads are not left unattended or in view of patients or other visitors to the office.

If a patient calls the office requesting a refill to be issued by the dentist, the office manager must inform the dentist of this request and note this on the patient's chart. Under no circumstances is she or he to issue (write or call in to the pharmacy) a refill for a prescription. Nor should the doctor sign blank prescriptions for use when she or he is away from the office. *Note:* Most dentists arrange for emergency coverage by another dentist in the area during extended planned absences from the office.

The Dental Laboratory Prescription

A sometimes overlooked record of the office is the dental **laboratory prescription.** When the dentist requires lab work done outside the office, the case must be sent with written instructions to be completed by the dental laboratory technician.

A dental lab prescription, sometimes referred to as a *work order,* is written in duplicate: one copy goes to the lab with the case and the other is retained in the patient's chart. The prescription's dual parts are usually labeled *"lab copy"* and *"office copy"* or *"doctor's copy."*

Many office managers find it helpful to set up a dental lab tracking system to enable the dentist and chairside assistant to know at any given time the location and status of every lab case sent out of the office.

This tracking system may be a notebook, a dry-wipe board in the office laboratory, or a tracking system logged into the computer data base (Figure 10-12). The tracking system should include:

Sample Lab Tracking Form					
Patient's Name	*Date Sent Out*	*Lab*	*Work Ordered*	*Date Needed*	*Patient's Appt.*
Mary Jones	10/3	Smile Dental	PFG 4-unit bridge	10/17	10/24
Harold Johnson	10/5	Dental Works	FU/FL Denture	10/12	11/3
Ralph Jenko	10/7	Dental Works	PU metal framework	10/18	10/20

Figure 10-12.   Sample lab tracking form.

It is also essential that the office manager keep a schedule of the required number of "turn-around" working days required by each respective lab to complete the procedure requested.

Note: The office manager must allow sufficient time when setting up appointments for the lab to complete the work and return it to the office prior to the patient's next scheduled appointment.

Most dental labs provide their own printed prescription pads for convenience. The following information should appear on the outgoing lab prescription:

- the patient's name (or sometimes a patient's case number)
- the type of service or prosthesis required

- the type of material required, such as porcelain or metal
- the shade (tooth color) required by the dentist to match the patient's original or existing dentition and a mould number for denture teeth
- the date required for the case to be returned to the office (usually one to two days prior to the patient's reappointment time)
- the dentist's name, address, telephone number, license number, and signature or initials

Note that a member of the dental staff may write dental lab work orders and sign the dentist's name or initials, as directed by the employer.

When the lab case is returned, it should be compared to the original work order or prescription for accuracy and quality. The returned case will include a copy of the prescription, which the office manager files to later compare to the monthly statements sent by the various labs with which the doctor works.

Skill-Building for Success: Student Activities

These optional activities and exercises are designed to help the student put into practice information learned in the chapter.

1. A patient of record is undergoing endodontic (root canal) treatment. She calls the office to request an additional refill of narcotic pain medication. The doctor is out of town for the next three business days. What are the office manager's options? How could she or he provide assistance to the patient and stay within legal guidelines? Divide into discussion groups and present at least three ideas to share with the class of how to handle this.

2. The dentist has directed that a young child with extensive decay should have two bitewing X-rays taken. The child is fearful, crying, and uncooperative; this is his first dental experience. The chairside assistant comes to you asking for your help. Divide into discussion groups and present at least three ideas to share with the class how this situation could be resolved.

3. Pretend you are the office manager calling to confirm all of tomorrow's patients. You notice that a patient is scheduled to have a four-unit bridge seated (cemented) tomorrow. You check the lab tracking system and discover the case is not back from the lab. What steps should you take? Divide into discussion groups and report at least three solutions to the class.

Skills Mastery Assessment: Post-Test

Directions: Select the response that *best* answers each of the following questions. Only one response is correct.

1. The complete patient file should contain the:
   a. first and last name of the patient
   b. clinical record, financial, and informed consent forms
   c. medical/dental history and necessary radiographs
   d. all of the above

2. Personal information or attributes about the patient should be included as part of the clinical or financial record.
   a. True
   b. False

3. Most practices conduct routine computer searches or manual audits of patient files to:
   a. keep patients from becoming lost in mid-treatment
   b. see that patients who may have canceled appointments without reappointing are rescheduled to complete treatment
   c. ensure that patients are notified of their recall appointments when due
   d. all of the above

4. It is the _____ job to contact and reschedule those patients who have incomplete treatment or who are past due for their recall appointments.
   a. dentist's
   b. sterilization assistant's
   c. office manager's
   d. dental hygienist's

5. Which of the following represents the correct alphabetical order?
   a. Hanson, P.; Hanson, Peter; Hanson, Peter Ralph
   b. Ward, John Henry; Ward, John H.; Mr. John Henry Ward
   c. McMullen, Cathryn; MacMullen, C.; McMullen, Sarah
   d. Garcia, J.J.; Garcia, Jose J.; Garcia, Jerry J.

6. The instructions "qid" to the pharmacist mean:
   a. four times a day
   b. every hour
   c. every four hours
   d. daily

7. A complete financial responsibility form should include all of the following *except:*
   a. the name, address, and phone number(s) of the patient and the responsible party (if different)
   b. specific insurance information such as the name of the carrier, the insured's group and/or policy number, and expiration date
   c. the patient's tax return from the previous year
   d. the responsible party's Social Security number and place of employment

8. The purpose of the medical health history is to alert the dentist to:
   a. prescribed drugs currently being taken by the patient
   b. current medical conditions and any known allergies
   c. the name and telephone number of a responsible party to contact in case of an emergency
   d. all of the above

9. When transferring patient records, the office manager should send legible, quality duplicates of the records—never the originals.
   a. True
   b. False

10. When forming a diagnosis, the dentist may require adjunct diagnostic aids including:
    a. dental radiographs (X-rays) or digital radiography
    b. periodontal disease susceptibility testing results
    c. study models and intraoral camera images
    d. all of the above

11. Periapical X-rays record the clinical crowns and interproximal areas of teeth and are used primarily for detection of carious lesions (decay) not visible to the naked eye.
    a. True
    b. False

12. Periapical films are used for all of the following except:
    a. diagnosis of periodontal disease
    b. subgingival and interproximal calculus
    c. sinus infections
    d. changes in pulpal health and abscesses

13. All of the following are true about panoramic X-rays *except:*
    a. the panoramic film is helpful to the dentist in detecting temporo-mandibular joint disorders and orthodontic conditions
    b. the panoramic film produces a somewhat enlarged image that is more diagnostically accurate than a full-mouth series
    c. the panoramic film is most often used in conjunction with a minimum of one set of posterior bitewing films
    d. the panoramic film is helpful in detecting impactions, supernumerary, and unerupted teeth

14. Radiation is *cumulative,* which means its effects dissipate quite rapidly.
    a. True
    b. False

15. Sometimes it is necessary for the operator to stand in the direct path of the X-ray beam to hold a film in a patient's mouth during exposure.
    a. True
    b. False

16. Which of the following are steps required to protect the patient during radiographic exposure?
    a. Place a protective lead apron with *thoracic* collar on all patients being exposed to radiation
    b. Take only the minimum number of films required by the dentist
    c. Use proper film positioning, exposure, and processing procedures to reduce the number of retakes
    d. all of the above

17. Benefits of digital radiography include:
    a. reduced radiation exposure for patients and dental team members
    b. reduced procedure exposure time and storage space
    c. enhanced diagnostic capability and high resolution with color-enhanced image quality
    d. all of the above

18. The periodontal disease predictability test uses a patient's blood sample to identify an excess amount of the disease-causing chemical that regulates the body's inflammatory response to bacteria.

   a. True
   b. False

19. The superscription is the portion of the prescription that contains the name of the drug, dosage form, and the amount of the dose.

   a. True
   b. False

20. All of the following information should appear on the outgoing lab prescription *except*:

   a. the shade (tooth color) required to match the patient's original or existing dentition
   b. the type of material required
   c. a copy of the patient's financial history form
   d. the date the prosthesis is required back in the office

References

Dietz, E. (1997). *Career enrichment: Expand the skills you have to create the job you want.* National Association of Dental Assistants.

Dietz, E. (1996). *Overcoming pitfalls of X-ray exposure and processing: A dental team approach.* [Home Study Program]. Woodland Hills, CA: Healthwatch.

(1996, September). Digital panoramic radiography using the DigiPan system by Trophy Radiology, Inc. *Dental Products Report.*

Expanding dental practice with computer technology. (1992). Princeton, NJ: Princeton Dental Resource Center.

Finkbeiner, B., & Johnson, C. (1995). *Mosby's comprehensive dental assisting: A clinical approach.* St. Louis: Mosby.

Genetic susceptibility to periodontal disease. [Brochure]. Flagstaff, AZ: Medical Science Systems, Inc.

Kross, J., DDS. (n.d.). Practice-building with intraoral cameras. *Progressive Dentistry.*

Vasquez, B., & Dennis, . (1997, Winter). Structure for good dental office-lab relationships. *Dental Economics Dental Equipment and Supplies.*

Weisman, G. (1996, March). Realistic expectation will help digital radiography contribute to the changing fact of dental practice. *Dental Products Report.*

Chapter 11

Scheduling to Optimize Practice Efficiency

- **Appointment Scheduling**
  Scheduling for the Dentist's Preference
  Scheduling to Meet Production Goals
  Blocking Out the Appointment Schedule
  Appointment Columns
  Multiple Appointments/Double-Booking
  Treatment Codes
  Scheduling Special-Needs Patients
- **Dental Emergency Patients**
  Screening and Scheduling Emergency Patients
  Screening Telephone Requests for Prescription Drugs
- **Recording Appointments**
  Sequential Appointment Scheduling
  Issuing the Patient's Appointment Card
- **Appointment Confirmation**
  Computerized Appointment Confirmation
- **Handling Late Patients**
  "No-show" Patients
  Maintaining a Call List
- **The Daily Schedule**
- **Scheduling Recall Appointments**
  Recall Appointment Confirmation
  Scheduling the Hygienist Who Works with an Assistant

Learning Objectives

Upon completion of this chapter, the student will achieve an 80 percent or higher score on the Skills Mastery Assessment Post-Test *covering the following material.*

1. List the priorities and considerations in scheduling appointments.
2. Describe the importance of time blocks/units in maintaining an efficient appointment system.
3. List the screening priorities of the office manager for handling and appointing emergency patients.
4. Describe scheduling considerations of special-needs patients.
5. Describe duties of the office manager when handling late patients and no-shows.
6. Describe the procedure for recording/scheduling appointments, completing appointment cards, and sequential appointment scheduling.
7. Describe the office manager's role in appointment confirmation and technology available to make confirmations.
8. Describe the importance of maintaining a patient call list.
9. List the office manager's duties in posting the daily schedule, maintaining the recall system, and scheduling the hygienist who works with an assistant.

Key Terms

block/unit appointment scheduling	palliative
call list	production scheduling
double-book	treatment codes

Appointment Scheduling

Scheduling is an essential business function of every successful dental practice. Some large practices employ staff members who only do scheduling, due to the importance of the role it plays in determining the profitability of the practice, the quality of the care provided, the emotional and physical well-being of the dentist and clinical staff, and the convenience and health of the patients.

Whether scheduling is completed manually in an appointment book or electronically on the computer, the same basic principles of scheduling apply. Scheduling should be week-at-a-glance and feature one column per operator's chair.

Scheduling for the Dentist's Preference

The first consideration in appointment scheduling is the dentist's energy level. Most practitioners prefer to perform demanding procedures, such as impactions, implants, and involved crown and bridge cases early in the day when they are most rested and alert. Oral surgery cases performed in the office under general anesthesia are scheduled early in the morning because they require the patient have nothing by mouth for eight hours preceding surgery.

Scheduling to Meet Production Goals

A second consideration in appointment scheduling is the practice's requirement to meet production goals in the form of cash flow. **Production-scheduling** decisions must follow the practice's strategies to generate adequate daily revenues to cover the overhead costs involved in running the practice, as well as to optimize profitability.

The office manager can meet these goals by scheduling more productive procedures first, and at times most convenient for patients, second. Thus, the office manager schedules for higher production figures first, then schedules the shorter or less productive visits in such a manner as not to rush or overburden the dental staff. Often, less complicated procedures can be staggered in between lengthier procedures to allow the patient several rest breaks throughout the procedure. For example, the dentist may leave the treatment room to conduct an oral examination on a hygiene patient or to inject the next patient scheduled for restorative treatment. In this way every patient receives courteous, attentive care and the practice sustains the resources necessary to offer excellent care soon after being seated.

A common example of scheduling that keeps both profitability and excellent care flowing consistently is multi-operatory scheduling that permits the dentist to see a follow-up patient or an adjustment patient while a patient who requires anesthesia is waiting for the injection to take effect. The patient is injected by the doctor, then monitored by the chairside assistant to ensure that there is no reaction. The dentist can see a patient for 5 or 10 minutes during this interval, return to prepare the anesthetized patient's tooth, then anesthetize a third patient while the assistant selects the shade for the first patient's completed prosthesis, prepares the adhesive and the temporary crown, waits for the impression material to set, removes the impression tray, and clears the patient's mouth of debris.

This interval provides sufficient time for the dentist to see another patient for a short visit, while the second patient's anesthetic takes effect.

Blocking Out the Appointment Schedule

Whether using the computer or a manual appointment book system, the office manager must plan ahead and block out specific times in which *not* to schedule patients. These times include lunch hours, holidays, the doctor's vacation/continuing education time away from the practice, buffer times for emergencies, and staff meetings. A sample computerized appointment schedule displays all the necessary components of electronic scheduling (Figure 11-1).

Appointment Columns

Dental appointments are scheduled in **blocks** or **units** of time, most often 10- or 15-minute units. This method optimizes the operator's time and helps keep everyone on staff on time as well.

If the dentist works on 15-minute time blocks and requests one hour for a crown preparation, impression, and temporization, the office manager reserves four units of the doctor's time in the primary column of the dentist's schedule or a total of four units. If the dentist prefers the 10-minute unit system, this same appointment would require six units of time.

To schedule efficiently, allowing neither too much nor too little time to complete procedures, the office manager must obtain from the dentist the

Appointment Book Window Areas

The Appointment Book window is divided into ten major areas: The Menu Bar, the Toolbar, the Time Bar, the Date Bar, the Calendar, the Arrow Buttons, the Schedule of Appointments, Pin Board, Flip Tabs, and the Day - Week - Month View Buttons.

Menu Bar

The Menu Bar provides the menu commands necessary to use all of the features provided as part of the Appointment Book.

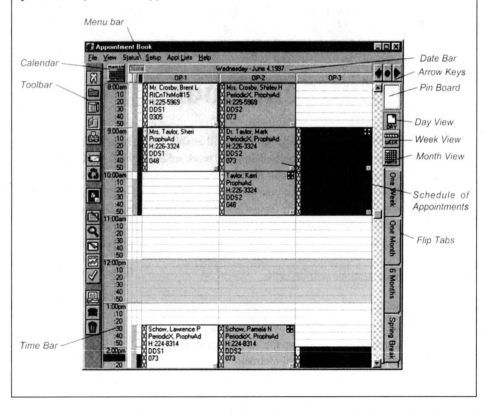

Figure 11-1. Sample electronic appointment book window. *(reprinted courtesy Dentrix Dental Systems, Inc. American Fork, UT.)*

desired number of appointment units for the most routinely performed procedures in the practice (Figure 11-2).

Appointment Units Required for Routine Procedures

Following is a sample list of time blocks used for routine dental appointments. Note that practices differ widely.

Type of Procedure	Amount of Time	10-Min. Units	15-Min. Units
Adult Prophylaxis	45–60 min.	4–5	3–4
Bonding Procedure	45–60 min.	4–5	3–4
Bridge Prep & Imp	(Depends upon number of units prepped) 45–90 min.	4–9	3–6
Child Prophylaxis	15–30 min.	2–3	2–3
Crown Prep & Imp	(Depends upon number of units prepped) 45–90 min.	4–9	3–6
Exam and Diagnosis	10–15 min.	1	1
Extraction	(Depends upon number of units and simplicity/ complexity of extractions) 30–90 min.	3–9	2–6
Implant Surgery	(Depends upon the number of units and complexity of case) 60–120 min.	6–12	4–8
Prosthesis Delivery	30–45 min.	3–4	2–3
Restorations	(Depends upon number of surfaces and quadrants involved) 30–60 min.	3–6	2–4
Root Canal Fill	45–60 min.	4–6	3–4

Figure 11-2.   Appointment units required for routine procedures.

Multiple Appointments/Double-Booking

Note that secondary appointments may be scheduled within an hour, such as post-operative checks for surgical patients, dental hygiene checks, and denture adjustments. The office manager may also schedule additional restorative patients and book them to arrive and be seated at staggered times. For example, the crown and bridge patient is scheduled for and seated at 10:00 a.m. The patient is greeted, seated, and anesthetized. At 10:15 the dentist checks the hygienist's 9:30 a.m. patient, whose prophylaxis has just been completed. This gives the anesthetic time to take effect on the patient seated in treatment room #1 and keeps the hygienist on schedule (Figure 11-3). Appointments are staggered throughout the day for optimal efficiency. Columns in the appointment schedule correspond to treatment room numbers utilized by operators.

Sample Portion of Appointment Book
with Multiple Columns and Staggered Scheduling

DENTIST COLUMN #1	DENTIST COLUMN #2	HYGIENIST
9:00 a.m. Quadrant restorative	9:45 a.m. Denture adj	9:30 a.m. Adult prophy
10:00 a.m. Seat and inject C & B Patient	10:15 a.m. Check Hyg.'s 9:30 adult prophy patient	10:30 a.m. Child prophy
10:45 a.m. Take C & B imp and have chairside asst. Make temporaries	10:30 a.m. Check Hyg.'s 10:30 prophy	11:00 a.m. Root planing & curettage
11:00 a.m. Check asst.'s temporaries and dismiss patient	11:10 a.m. Inject next patient and seat 3-unit bridge; conclude at 12:00 and check hyg.'s root planing & curettage patient	Conclude at 12:00

Figure 11-3. Sample portion of appointment book with multiple columns and staggered scheduling.

Multiple appointment columns also work effectively in double-booking appointments, that is, in scheduling patients who are chronically late, who have a history of disappointment (not showing), or for scheduling emergencies.

Treatment Codes

Because many practices accept some form of third-party coverage toward payment for services, the office manager may be requested to include the corresponding **treatment code** adjacent to each procedure scheduled (Figure 11-4) to track and facilitate payment properly. Treatment codes are assigned by individual insurance carriers; most practices utilize the treatment codes established by the American Dental Association.

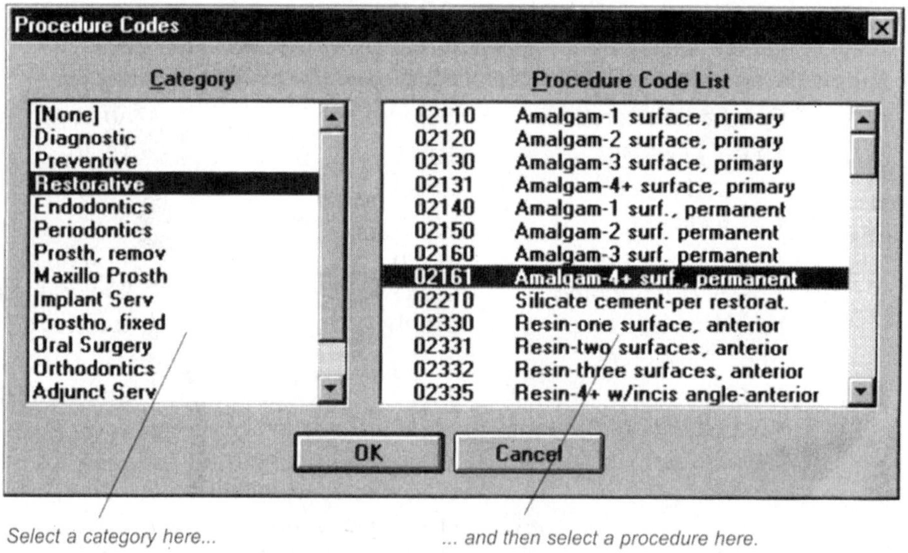

Figure 11-4. Sample procedure codes used for appointment scheduling and subsequent third-party billing. *(reprinted courtesy Dentrix Dental Systems, Inc. American Fork, UT.)*

Scheduling Special-Needs Patients

Patients having special needs may require additional appointment blocks. Special-needs patients include, but are not limited to, known dental phobics, hyperactive children, patients with bleeding disorders, physically or mentally handicapped individuals, elderly patients who require assistance, patients with heart conditions, patients who require premedication for management of anxiety or prevention of bacterial endocarditis, and patients who require general anesthesia or conscious sedation. Patients covered under the *Americans with Disabilities Act* may also have special needs.

The office manager should check with the dentist before scheduling special-needs patients as to the additional time required for preoperative, operative, and postoperative considerations. In cases of severe mental retardation or other physical limitations, the dentist may prefer to admit the patient to the hospital for treatment under general anesthesia or to refer the patient to a specialist who has hospital privileges.

Elderly patients, homemakers, and retired patients who are available during daytime hours should be scheduled to fill times during the day that are most difficult to fill. Young children should be scheduled for morning appointments as they are at a lowered activity level and generally more cooperative. Diabetic patients should be scheduled early in the morning when their insulin levels tend to be more stable.

Dental Emergency Patients

Few patients actually experience true dental emergencies. (An emergency is characterized as severe trauma, such as that resulting from an automobile accident or other injury or an accidental tooth avulsion—a tooth knocked out of the socket—or jaw fracture.) In most true dental emergency situations, patients are taken to the hospital emergency room for treatment and/or referral to an oral surgeon or other specialist. Occasionally, however, individuals call the office requiring treatment related to pain, swelling, or a lost or broken prosthesis or restoration.

Most practices are committed to treating all emergency patients, regardless of inconvenience to the dentist or the patient's ability to pay.

In most practices, emergency visits are **palliative** only, which means the dentist treats only the immediate source of the pain or nature of the problem (such as recementing a crown) and reappoints the patient at another time for a complete examination, diagnosis, and treatment plan. Usually only an *Emergency Treatment Form* is created for emergency patients; however, the treatment is thoroughly documented.

Screening and Scheduling Emergency Patients

Emergency patients must be screened by the office manager to determine the following: 1) whether the caller is a patient of record; 2) the extent, onset, and severity of the symptoms; 3) other related circumstances (Figure 11-5).

Some practices have a specific (buffer) time reserved in their daily schedules to accommodate routine emergencies. These times are often just before

---

Screening Emergency Callers Who Request Treatment

The office manager may use the following questions to obtain additional information and screen emergency callers:

- Are you a patient of record with the practice? (Ask this only if unfamiliar with the patient's name.)
- Please describe the symptoms/nature of the emergency.
- How long have the pain and/or swelling been present? (Ask only if pain and/or swelling are reported by the caller.)
- Is the discomfort constant? Does it keep you up at night?
- Does the discomfort increase in response to any of the following: heat, cold, sweets, or pressure?
- Is the caller presently under the care of a physician for other medical conditions or taking prescription medications? If so, what types and dosages?
- Does the caller have known drug allergies or sensitivities to prescription medications?

Figure 11-5.   Screening emergency callers who request treatment.

or after the lunch hour or at the end of the day. Other practices prefer to handle dental emergency calls at the direction of the dentist.

Screening Telephone Requests for Prescription Drugs

In some instances, known or suspected drug abusers may call the office in pain, requesting prescriptions for narcotics. The wise office manager alerts the dentist to possible drug abusers "shopping" for pain medication. The conscientious dentist is very careful *not* to provide prescription drugs to individuals who might abuse or resell controlled substances. Some states now require *separate* prescriptions to be written specifically for narcotics.

At the decision of the dentist, an emergency patient may be given a prescription for an antibiotic if an infection must be brought under control prior to initiating a corrective procedure.

Recording Appointments

Upon request to schedule an appointment and with the knowledge of the necessary procedure and number of time units required, the office manager determines a time of preference for the patient. A significant key to practice building is providing availability of convenient appointment times for patients.

Rather than simply assigning an appointment time, some practices ask patients on the *New Patient Registration Form* for their preference of convenient appointment times. Other practices pick two open times in the appointment schedule and offer the patient a choice. For example, "Mrs. Jones, I understand you prefer early morning appointments. Would 9:00 a.m. on Tuesday, March the 7, or 8:30 a.m. on Thursday, March 9th be more convenient?" This gives the patient a sense of convenience and control over the appointment schedule. Patients also like to be given choices, where possible, rather than being assigned one specific time only.

Whether using a manual appointment book or electronic scheduling, it is imperative that the office manager record the patient's name, appointment time, number of units, and abbreviation of the procedure scheduled. When using a manual system, a line or arrow is drawn through the total number of appointment units required to allow sufficient time to complete the procedure. If, for example, a new adult patient is to be scheduled for a one-hour prophylaxis appointment and necessary radiographs with the hygienist, the office manager writes the patient's name in the hygienist's column of the appointment schedule next to the appointed time (9:00 a.m.), along with the notation, "NP/PX" and draws a line or an arrow through all the time slots up until 10:00 a.m. This indicates that no other appointments are to be scheduled in that time block. Note that the office manager should record the appointment time in the book or on the computer scheduling data base first, then complete an appointment card, if the patient is present in the office at the time of scheduling. This is to avoid the embarrassment of a patient's presenting for treatment only to discover that another appointment was scheduled at the same time.

Sequential Appointment Scheduling

When a series or sequence of planned treatments is indicated, some dentists prefer that the patient be scheduled for all appointments at the outset of treatment. This helps keep planned treatment on schedule and prevents patients from becoming lost in the system throughout the phase of treatment. In such cases, the dentist should indicate the number of appointments, the number of units to be blocked for each, and the anticipated treatment to take place during that appointment.

The wise office manager notes that when outside laboratory work is required on a case, sufficient time must be allotted to allow the case to be sent out, fabricated, and returned in time for the patient's next scheduled visit.

When patients are scheduled for multiple appointments, some offices also set up payment schedules to correspond to the planned treatment visits for patients to pay-as-they-go. This helps the patient to schedule appointments according to his or her financial obligations and also informs him or her of all anticipated treatment costs prior to the appointment. (This pre-estimation helps avoid financial surprises and gives the patient a clear plan of planned treatment and his or her financial responsibility.)

Issuing the Patient's Appointment Card

If the patient is present during the appointment scheduling, the office manager provides an appointment card containing the date(s) of the scheduled appointment(s) and the name of the operator with whom he or she is appointed, as well as the date, time, and day of the week. A notice usually appears at the bottom of the appointment card requesting that any change in appointment be requested 24 hours in advance. While some practices charge for broken or missed appointments, most do not. For further information on completing appointment cards, see *Chapter 6, Printed Communications.*

Appointment Confirmation

Once an appointment or series of appointments has been established it becomes vital that the office manager contact patients to confirm their scheduled appointments. This most often occurs the day before the appointment via a telephone call. Office managers find early mornings and later afternoon and evenings the most effective time to reach patients at home to confirm their appointments.

The office manager creates the next day's set of scheduled appointments on a *daily schedule*, a copy of which is posted in each treatment room. From the day schedule she or he pulls the files (if the practice is on a manual system) and from these calls patients to confirm their appointments. As patients are reached and their appointments confirmed, the office manager makes a check mark or other visual indicator that the patient has been reached and/or that a message has been left.

Patients who list a daytime telephone number other than their homes, usually their work, office, mobile phone, car phone, or pager number, may also be contacted during the workday to confirm appointments. The conversation is brief and to the point and may be as follows, "Hello, Mr. Daniels, this is Mary calling from Dr. Edwards' office. I'm calling to confirm your 9:30 a.m. appointment tomorrow." The patient is then given the opportunity to respond.

Some patients are difficult to reach and the office manager may leave a message on their voice messaging or personal answering machine. On occasion when the patient cannot be contacted, the office manager may take home a list of those patients who could not be reached for confirmation and will call them later in the evening. This is at the dentist's direction.

Computerized Appointment Confirmation

Some technologically more advanced offices use computerized or automated appointment confirmation systems. The office computer dials the numbers of the appointed patients and plays a prerecorded message such as, "This is Shannon at Dr. Olsen's office, with an important confirmation message. According to our records, we will be treating a member of your household in our office tomorrow. We want to confirm with you that this time is currently reserved especially for your appointed procedure. If you have questions about your appointment, please call Shannon at (_____ number)."

Technological time-savers help free an hour or two of the office manager's time to focus on face-to-face relationships with patients as they present for treatment.

Note: An autodialer can provide a routine memory-jogger for practice personnel to make more important calls to patients who require extra attention; however, it cannot take the place of sound patient relations skills. Similarly, learning to utilize a sophisticated communication system incorporating telephone, fax, computerized dental office management, and possibly computer-aided clinical diagnosis is not an end in itself. These tools are as powerful as the user makes them, but they are only the means to mastering patient and interoffice communications. Successful communication has always been and will always be an interpersonal skill.

Handling Late Patients

Occasionally, patients cannot help being detained and thus arrive late for their appointments. Unfortunately, this may require the necessity to either reschedule the patient, provide less than the planned time for treatment that day to keep on schedule, or to delay subsequent patients' treatment.

Some offices make a habit of recognizing patients who chronically arrive late for appointments and either schedule them later in the day or inform them that their appointments are 10 or 15 minutes earlier than actually scheduled. Another option is to **double-book** chronically late patients to keep the practice and patient flow running smoothly. The office manager should note and initial in the chart any late arrival behavior and the date.

"No-Show" Patients

Patients who fail to keep confirmed appointments are commonly referred to as *no-shows*. Failing to keep an appointment is sometimes called a *disappointment.* Practices that experience a high rate of no-shows or disappointments often require a review of their scheduling and appointment confirmation procedures.

The office manager should note and initial all no-shows or disappointments in the patient's chart with the date.

Maintaining a Call List

A **call list** is a handy reference for the office manager to fill an opening in the appointment schedule on short notice. Some especially busy practices or those that have a long waiting period for appointments provide a space on their *New Patient Registration Form* that asks patients if they are available on short notice and if they would like to be placed on a call list to be contacted on short notice should an opening in the schedule occur.

The call list may be a manually written sheet or notebook of patients desiring to be contacted on short notice for required treatment to be completed; it can also be maintained on the office computer. The following information should be included on the call list: the date the patient was added to the call list, the name of the patient, the type of procedure needed, the required number of appointment units and the daytime telephone number. Note that once a patient has been contacted and appointed earlier in the schedule, his or her name should be: 1) removed from the call list to avoid future embarrassment of being called to provide a procedure that has already been completed, and 2) removed from the original appointment book or computer scheduling program.

When an opening occurs in the schedule on short notice, the office manager should always start with the top of the call list, reviewing patients in the chronological order of their placement on the list. This avoids the potential for favoritism and treats all patients on the call list fairly.

The Daily Schedule

The office manager maintains the daily schedule based upon the appointment book or computerized program. It is the office manager's responsibility to see that scheduling is carried out to the dentist's preference, to meet production goals and to accommodate patients' schedules.

Each day a copy of the daily schedule is posted in each treatment room, usually late the prior afternoon, for the dentist(s), hygienist(s), and chairside assistants to review. This brings them up to date on which patients are scheduled, which patients' appointments have been confirmed, and alerts them to raise concerns or ask questions early the next day at the morning huddle (Figure 11-6).

Occasionally, changes in the daily schedule occur. It is the office manager's job to note these changes on the daily schedule and to alert the operators to these schedule changes.

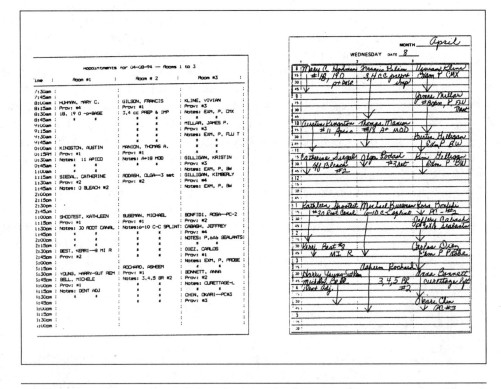

Figure 11-6.   Examples of daily schedules, both computer-generated and handwritten.

Scheduling Recall Appointments

Recall appointments are addressed in several areas throughout this text. The wise office manager knows that recall appointments are a vital lifeline in sustaining the growth and productivity of the practice. Many practices set specific recall goals for scheduling returning patients. Most dental practice management authorities agree that an 85 percent return rate of recall patients scheduled is successful.

Recall Appointment Confirmation

The office manager handles and confirms recall (sometimes referred to as *recare*) appointments in the same manner as the doctor's appointments. Charts are pulled the day prior, from the appointment book or computer program; a day sheet is compiled listing the names and appointed times patients are scheduled, and the type of procedure anticipated. The office manager calls the patients to confirm their appointments.

Once the hygienist has completed the patient's recall appointment, the office manager either reschedules the patient for the next due recall appointment (or enters the date for the next recall notification into the computer or manual recall filing system). If the patient requires restorative treatment, the office manager sets up the required series of appointments for the patient to return to be treated by the dentist.

Scheduling the Hygienist Who Works with an Assistant

In some practices the hygienist works with an assistant who provides chairside services not specifically delegated only to the hygienist. This helps the hygienist work more efficiently and makes the practice more productive. Of course, this is also dependent upon the individual practice act of the state of employment and the permitted duties of assistants.

The office manager schedules the hygienist's time for such procedures as subgingival scaling, deep scaling, curettage, administration of local anesthesia and/or conscious sedation, and suture removal. The office manager may schedule the hygienist's assistant to provide such services as completion or updating of necessary forms, oral radiography procedures, operatory set-up and clean-up, instrument preparation and sterilization, coronal polish, pit and fissure sealant application, topical fluoride application, and oral hygiene instruction.

In such practices the hygienist usually works back and forth between two treatment rooms while the hygiene assistant is in the other room with the second hygiene patient. The hygiene scheduling flow may function as follows (Figure 11-7):

***Sample Description of Work Flow
of Hygienist Working with an Assistant***

8:00 a.m.

Hygiene assistant seats and drapes adult recall patient and updates medical history; opens sterile instrument pack in front of patient; exposes bitewing X-rays and excuses him/herself to load films into automatic processor and set up the adjacent hygiene treatment room for next patient.

8:15 a.m.

Hygienist enters the treatment room and performs oral cancer screening exam, proceeds with recording periodontal scores and performing deep scaling procedure.

8:45 a.m.

Hygiene assistant returns to the treatment room with patient's films mounted and places them on the viewbox for the hygienist and dentist to review. Dentist enters room to conduct oral exam.

Dentist and hygienist excuse themselves and hygiene assistant concludes the patient's visit with a coronal polish. The dentist returns to an operative procedure and the hygienist moves to the adjacent hygiene operatory to inject the next patient for deep scaling and curettage.

At conclusion of hygiene appointment, the hygiene assistant dismisses patient, informs the office manager of the patient's subsequent scheduling needs, and returns to the treatment room for clean-up, removal of contaminated instruments, room disinfection, replacing of protective barriers, and other procedures required to ready the treatment room for the next patient.

Figure 11-7. Sample description of work flow of hygienist working with an assistant.

Thus, scheduling for efficiency and productivity is a key responsibility of the office manager. Possessing skills of appointment schedule management are essential in assuming an office management position.

Skill-Building for Success: Student Activities

These optional activities and exercises are designed to help the student put into practice information learned in the chapter.

1. You are a new office manager in a large urban setting. A caller with whom you are unfamiliar says he has been in pain with a bad toothache for 24 hours. What actions should you take? What questions should you ask? Make a list of steps you would take and then take turns sharing your answers with the class.

2. You arrive at 8:30 a.m. on Monday as the new office manager to discover that two patients have been inadvertently scheduled for the same appointment time with the dentist. What should you do? Make a list of possible solutions and take turns sharing your ideas with the class.

Skills Mastery Assessment: Post-Test

Directions: Select the response that *best* answers each of the following questions. Only one response is correct.

1. What considerations must be taken into account when scheduling for productivity?

   a. the time of day preferred by the dentist to perform the procedure
   b. the daily cash flow requirements of the practice
   c. the impact of scheduling decisions on patient flow
   d. all the above

2. Ethical dentists offer complete restorative treatment to all emergency patients regardless of their ability to pay.

   a. True
   b. False

3. Which of the following information should be included on the call list?

   a. the date the patient was added to the call list
   b. the type of procedure needed, days and hours available
   c. the required number of appointment units
   d. all of the above

4. Times blocked out of the appointment schedule usually include all of the following *except:*

   a. lunch hours
   b. holidays
   c. visits from dental supply representatives
   d. buffer times for emergencies and staff meetings

5. Appointment blocks or units of time are most often in _____ increments:

   a. 1- or 2-hour
   b. 10- or 15-minute
   c. 15- or 30-minute
   d. varying

6. Double-booking is a scheduling technique used to:

   a. manage habitually late or no-show patients
   b. maximize the doctor's time efficiently
   c. save space in the appointment book
   d. a and b only

7. Treatment codes are assigned to each procedure to facilitate third-party payment.
   a. True
   b. False

8. Special-needs patients who may require adjustments in time units scheduled include:
   a. those covered under the *Americans with Disabilities Act*
   b. patients who require premedication for management of anxiety or prevention of bacterial endocarditis
   c. patients who require general anesthesia
   d. all of the above

9. Few patients actually experience true dental emergencies.
   a. True
   b. False

10. What is the proper sequence for scheduling and confirming an appointment?
    a. make out the appointment card, call the day before to confirm the appointment, record the appointment in the book or computer database
    b. call the day before to confirm the appointment, make out the appointment card, record the appointment in the book or computer database
    c. record the appointment in the book or computer database, make out the appointment card, call the day before to confirm the appointment
    d. There is no set way to schedule and confirm appointments.

11. Early mornings and later afternoon and evenings are the most effective time to reach patients at home to confirm their appointments.
    a. True
    b. False

12. An auto-dialer provides a routine memory-jogger for practice personnel to make more important calls to patients who require extra attention and replaces sound patient relations skills.
    a. True
    b. False

13. The daily schedule:
    a. is posted in each treatment room, usually late the prior afternoon
    b. brings all clinical personnel up to date on which patients are scheduled and confirmed for the next day
    c. alerts staff to raise concerns or ask questions early the next day at the morning huddle
    d. all of the above

14. Young children should be scheduled for late appointments when they are at a lowered activity level and are generally more cooperative.

    a. True
    b. False

15. Diabetic patients should be scheduled early in the morning when their insulin levels are more stable.

    a. True
    b. False

16. Some practices have a specific (buffer) time reserved in their daily schedules to accommodate routine emergencies. These times are often:

    a. just before or after the lunch hour
    b. at the end of the day
    c. whenever the patient can come in to the office
    d. a or b only

17. Having an assistant helps the hygienist work more efficiently and makes the practice more productive.

    a. True
    b. False

18. The office manager schedules the hygienist's time for such procedures as:

    a. subgingival scaling
    b. deep scaling and curettage
    c. administration of local anesthesia and/or conscious sedation and suture removal
    d. all of the above procedures

References

Blatchford, W. (1990, February). Block scheduling for results. *Dentistry Today*.

Griffin, A. P. Analysis of current activities in the practice. Greenville, NC: Practicon, Inc.

Chapter 12

Managing Accounts Receivable

- **Managed Care Programs**
  - Health Maintenance Organizations (HMOs)
  - Preferred Provider Organizations (PPOs)
  - Exclusive Provider Organizations (EPOs)
  - Point-of-Service Plans (POSs)
- **Insurance and Third-party Claims Processing**
  - Terminology and Procedures
  - The Standard (ADA) Claim Form
- **ADA Insurance Codes**
  - Predetermination and Preauthorization
  - Signature on File
  - Walk-out Statement
  - Use of Digital Radiographs and Intraoral Photographs
- **The One-Write System**
- **Electronic Claims Processing**
- **Claims Tracking and Rejection**
- **Methods of Payment**
  - Cash and Cash Discounts
  - Personal Check
  - Private Label Dental Care Cards
  - Credit Cards and Credit/Debit Card Readers
  - Direct Reimbursement
  - Series of Payments
  - Cycle Billing
  - The Typical Billing/Collection Cycle
  - Finance Plans
- **Procedure for Entering a Payment**
- **Performing a Credit Check**

• **Collection of Past-due Accounts**
    Collection Telephone Calls
    Small Claims Court and Collection Agencies

Learning Objectives

Upon completion of this chapter, the student will achieve an 80 percent or higher score on the Skills Mastery Assessment Post-Test *covering the following material.*

1. Define managed care and describe alternative payment plans with regard to the dental practice.
2. Describe and define insurance and other third-party payment claims processing and related terminology; complete a standard insurance form accurately.
3. Describe the use and components of a one-write system.
4. Describe the benefits of electronic claims processing.
5. Describe methods of patient payment for dental treatment.
6. Describe the procedure for entering payments.
7. Explain the procedure and rationale for performing a credit check.
8. Describe the procedure for collection of past due accounts.

Key Terms

capitation	electronic claims processing
coordination of benefits	insured party
copayment	managed care
costs of credit	provider
credit check	responsible party
direct reimbursement	signature on file
dual coverage	walk-out statement

Managed Care Programs

Managed care involves any third party's participation in the management of healthcare delivery with regard to finance. It includes predetermination of benefits and claims reviews, as well as fully managed **capitation** programs. Patients who enroll in managed care choose a specific participating office according to a list of dentists who enroll and agree to the managed care company's terms. The office is then responsible for all of the general, and in some cases specialty, dental services required.

Managed care is a cost-containment system that directs the utilization of health benefits by limiting the type, level, and frequency of treatment; limiting access to care; and controlling the level of reimbursement for services.

The primary advantage for a dentist to sign up for a managed care program is a guaranteed flow of new patients. Another advantage is that administrative costs are minimized because there are no claims to process, there is a guaranteed cash flow, and a guaranteed patient base (number of patients). This is especially appealing to a new dentist just starting out in practice or trying to build a practice.

A primary disadvantage for the dentist participating in a capitation-based program is that the risk for utilization of services by patients beyond that anticipated falls on the dentist instead of on the insurance company.

Following are descriptions of the main types of managed care organizations.

Health Maintenance Organizations (HMOs)

Health Maintenance Organizations (HMOs) are broken down into four types: *staff models, group models, Individual Practice Associations (IPAs)* and *network models.*

The classic HMO is the *staff model,* in which the healthcare plan owns the facility and pays **providers** (dentists) to work in them. In this type of plan patients are restricted to the HMO's providers (doctors and hospitals) and must seek treatment from primary caregivers before being referred to specialists. About 10 percent of all HMOs are staff model.

The *group model* is a variation on the staff model. In the group model the HMO contracts with an individual provider group to care for its patients. The provider group is managed independently and reimbursed on a capitated basis. Capitation refers to a method of payment for services where the insurer pays providers a fixed amount for each patient treated, regardless of the type, complexity, or number of services required. About 10 percent of all HMOs are group model.

Individual Practice Associations (IPAs) are the most common type of HMO, comprising 65 percent of all plans. IPAs contract either with individual providers or with networks of providers who practice in their own offices. Some providers and networks are paid discounted fee-for-service; however many are capitated.

The fourth type of HMO is the *network model,* which comprises approximately 15 percent of dental managed care plans. It is similar to the IPA model because it forms a network of independent provider groups, which may be single-specialty or multi-specialty. Providers in the network model may be paid by either discounted fee-for-service or capitation and may continue to provide services to their own private patients.

Preferred Provider Organizations (PPOs)

Under a *Preferred Provider Organization (PPO)* a third-party (an insurer, an employer, administrator, or other sponsoring group) negotiates discounted rates for dental services directly with selected provider dentists. *Beneficiaries* (those eligible or enrolled patients in the plan) covered by the PPO may use providers outside the PPO network, although financial incentives encourage patients to use preferred providers. Providers in a PPO are selected based upon their professional qualifications and performance; they benefit through increased patient volume and prompt payment. In return, providers agree to a fee schedule and review of their performance.

Exclusive Provider Organizations (EPOs)

Exclusive Provider Organizations (EPOs) evolved from PPOs. The EPO is an indemnity arrangement where a group of providers contracts with an insurer, third-party administrator, employer, or other sponsor. The provider agrees to accept the negotiated level of reimbursement, to follow utilization review procedures (audits), to refer patients to other EPO-contracted providers, and to use only contracted hospitals (when a patient requires hospitalization, for example for full-mouth extractions under general anesthesia).

In contrast with a PPO, the EPO provider can be prohibited from treating patients not enrolled in the organization. Patients (beneficiaries) must seek services only from participating providers. In an EPO any dental services provided by unaffiliated providers are not reimbursed.

Point-of-Service Plans (POSs)

Members of a *Point-of-Service Plan (POS)* receive care from participating providers designated by the network, but have the option of obtaining care outside the network. Both HMOs and PPOs may offer a POS plan as a method of expanding members' options of providers. These agreements are called "open-ended." If a member receives treatment from a provider who is not a part of the network, the care is covered, although it will likely include a high **copayment.** (The amount the patient pays at the time of service for treatment.)

Insurance and Third-party Claims Processing

Payment options often include insurance participation. In fact, approximately 60 percent of all dental practices accept and/or participate in some form of insurance or *third-party* coverage for their patients who have coverage. (Third-party means a party, other than the dentist or the patient, is involved in financial responsibility for treatment.)

It is the dental office manager's responsibility to complete and submit insurance claim forms. Some practices, especially large groups, employ a staff member who deals exclusively with insurance claims processing.

Many patients who have obtained dental insurance for the first time have the misconception that their dental care is covered completely by insurance. To avoid misunderstandings at the outset it is the office manager's duty to explain that usually only a certain percentage of the total fee is covered (allowed) by the insurance company and ultimately it is the patient's responsibility to pay the remaining portion. (While "sold" as a benefit of employment, most dental insurance plans cover only a portion of treatment required.)

For example, the insurance provider may agree to pay 50 percent of a restorative procedure, not to exceed $350 for a porcelain-fused-to-metal crown. Thus, if the dentist's fee for the crown is $650 and the insurance company pays the first $350, the patient is responsible for paying the remaining $300 at the time the crown is seated. Under managed care, the dentist receives only the $350.

Terminology and Procedures

An important step to successful completion of this task is obtaining and reporting complete third-party information. This includes obtaining all necessary information including the name of the **insured party,** the **responsible party** (if not the same), spouse, parent, or guardian of the insured party; plus the names of the employer, employer code or group number, the address and telephone number for submitting claims, and the acceptable method(s) for claims submission(s) (Figure 12-1).

Some insurance companies allow for **coordination of benefits** when the patient is covered by more than one carrier or policy, as in the case of working spouses, both of whom carry dental insurance, and/or their children, who are covered under both plans. In this circumstance the dentist bills the *primary* insurance provider first, then sends the same claim to the *secondary* provider to pay the allowable benefit on the remaining unpaid balance. (Rarely, however is treatment covered 100 percent by both plans.)

When both insurance carriers participate this is termed **dual coverage.** It requires further research by the office manager to ensure that coordination of benefits is permitted and the extent to which both carriers provide coverage (i.e., the dollar amount or percentage).

Dependent children of dual coverage parents are covered as "primary" by the plan of the respective parent whose birthday falls earlier in the calendar year. Dependent children with divorced or legally separated parents are covered according to the following guidelines:

1. The biological parent who has custody.
2. The spouse of the biological parent who has custody.
3. The non-custodial biological parent.
4. The spouse of the non-custodial biological parent.
5. If the terms of the divorce decree place financial obligation on one parent, that parent's insurance is primary over the secondary plan.

Attending Dentist's Statement

Check one:
☐ Dentist's pre-treatment estimate
☒ Dentist's statement of actual services

Carrier name and address
Dental Care Insurance Company
1500 Western Avenue
Middleton, CA 98765

PATIENT SECTION

1. Patient name first / m.i. / last	2. Relationship to employee	3. Sex	4. Patient birthdate MM DD YYYY	5. If full time student
Jason P. Rangers	X self ☐ child ☐ spouse ☐ other	x	11 24 1950	

6. Employee/subscriber name and mailing address
Self
2356 Harmony Avenue
Prospect, CA 98766

7. Employee/subscriber soc. sec. number
111-22-3333

8. Employee/subscriber birthdate MM DD YYYY
11 24 1950

9. Employer (company) name and address
Sanders Refuse
14th&Main Sts.
Prospect, CA

10. Group number
4590

11. Is patient covered by another plan of benefits?
Dental none
Medical health

12-a. Name and address of carrier(s)
Maxima Health Ins.

12-b. Group no.(s)
2847B

13. Name and address of employer
none

14-a. Employee/subscriber name (if different than patient's)

14-b. Employee/subscriber soc. sec. number
same

14-c. Employee/subscriber birthdate MM DD YYYY
--

15. Relationship to patient
X self ☐ parent ☐ spouse ☐ other

I have reviewed the following treatment plan. I authorize release of any information relating to this claim. I understand that I am responsible for all costs of dental treatment.

► *Jason P. Rangers* 8-15xx
Signed (Patient, or parent if minor) / Date

I hereby authorize payment directly to the below named dentist of the group insurance benefits otherwise payable to me.

► *Jason P. Rangers* 8/15/xx
Signed (Insured person) / Date

DENTIST SECTION

16. Dentist name
Jay V. School

17. Mailing address
5600 Professional Building SuiteD
Prospect, CA 98766

18. Dentist Soc. Sec. or T.I.N.
999-88-7777

19. Dentist license no.
CA8476

20. Dentist phone no.
302-555-1111

21. First visit date current series
8/1/xx

22. Place of treatment
Office x

24. Is treatment result of occupational illness or injury?	No	Yes	If yes, enter brief description and dates.
	X		
25. Is treatment result of auto accident?	X		
26. Other accident?	X		
27. Are any services covered by another plan?		X	
28. If prosthesis, is this initial placement?			(If no, reason for replacement) / 29. Date of prior placement
30. Is treatment for orthodontics?	X		If services already commenced enter: / Date appliances placed / Mos. treatment remaining

23. Radiographs or models enclosed? No Yes How many? x

31. Examination and treatment plan - List in order from tooth no. 1 through tooth no. 32 - Use charting system shown.

Tooth # or letter	Surface	Description of service (including x-rays, prophylaxis, materials used, etc.) Line No.	Date service performed Mo. Day Year	Procedure number	Fee	For administrative use only
		1 oral examination	08 01xx 0	0120	24 00	
		2 Bite wing radiographs(2)	08 01xx 0	2720	16 00	
		3 Prophylaxis	08 01xx 0	1110	32 00	
8	M	4 Composite restoration 1 sur	08 15xx 0	2330	44 00	
18	MO	5 Amalgam restoration 2 sur	08 15xx 0	2150	48 00	
		6				
		7				
		8				
		9				
		10				
		11				
		12				
		13				
		14				
		15				

32. Remarks for unusual services

I hereby certify that the procedures as indicated by date have been completed and that the fees submitted are the actual fees I have charged and intend to collect for those procedures.
Date 8/16/xx
Signed (Dentist)

Total Fee Charged	164 00
Max. Allowable	
Deductible	
Carrier %	
Carrier pays	
Patient pays	

Form approved by the
American Dental Association
(ADS 85)
#29375 · Medical Arts Press 1 800 328 2179

Figure 12-1. Sample dental insurance form completed and ready for submission. *(provided courtesy of Medical Arts Press 1-800-328-2179.)*

If the dentist participates in a program with *usual, customary and reasonable fee (UCR),* she or he files the UCR fees with the carrier. Payment is based upon the percentage covered by the group.

If the dentist participates in a *fixed fee* program, this means a fixed fee has been predetermined for every allowable procedure. Dentists who participate in fixed fee programs must accept the fees established and are not legally allowed to charge the patient the additional amount for the balance.

Each insurance carrier provides a *table of allowance,* which establishes a fixed dollar amount for each patient's dental services. In this case the patient is financially responsible for any difference between the fee charged by the dentist and the table amount.

Benefit refers to the amount the insurance company pays toward services covered under the contractual plan. *Carrier* refers to the company that sells or carries insurance. *Coverage* refers to the extent of the insurance policy (i.e., the benefits included). *Deductible* refers to the amount the patient or responsible party must pay toward services before the carrier will begin paying on insurance claims. *Exclusions* refers to services not covered under the terms of the policy.

The Standard (ADA) Claim Form

The following information is required when completing a third-party insurance claim form. Missing or incomplete information may cause a delay in payment or trigger the claim to be rejected. The office manager must ensure the following information is completed and reported on every insurance claim form (Figure 12-2).

Whether filing manually or electronically, the office manager makes sure one copy is in the patient's financial record and another goes to the insurance company.

ADA Insurance Codes

Third-party reimbursement processing requires the use of treatment codes when claims are submitted for payment. This is to ensure that each procedure is properly billed and that the correct amount is paid to the provider. Procedures for which no code is provided are usually not reimbursed.

Insurance Information Required to Submit A Claim

- The dentist's pretreatment estimate (used when extensive treatment is planned) or actual statement of services provided
- The carrier's name and address
- The patient's legal name
- The patient's relationship to the employee (if different)
- The patient's gender
- The patient's date of birth
- Notation of the patient's full-time student status (if applicable)
- The employee/subscriber's name (this is the insured person)
- The employee's name
- The employee/subscriber's social security number
- The employee/subscriber's mailing address
- The name of the group dental plan
- The location of the union local or number
- Whether the patient is covered by any other dental plan
- The dentist's social security number or tax identification number (TIN)
- The dentist's license number
- The dentist's telephone number with area code
- The date of the first visit
- Whether radiographs, study models, or other related diagnostic aids are included with the claim submission
- Place the treatment or service was rendered
- The result of treatment; whether the treatment was necessitated by an automobile accident
- Date of initial placement (if a prosthesis is required)
- If the treatment required is orthodontic in nature
- Results of the examination and treatment plan
- The insured person's signature
- The dentist's name, address and signature

Figure 12-2. Insurance information required to submit a claim.

The American Dental Association publishes a book (*CDT-2*) containing an extensive list, by category and treatment, of dental and related procedures. The book is updated every five years. The office manager should keep a current copy at the front desk for easy access.

Many office managers prefer to make up a shortened list of the practice's most commonly used insurance codes, either by alphabetical or numerical listing. This saves valuable time when preparing and submitting claims (see *Chapter 9, Charting the Oral Cavity* for further information on insurance codes).

Predetermination and Preauthorization

Many insurance carriers require requests to perform procedures be filed in advance. *Predetermination* means the amount or percentage the insurance company agrees to pay toward the total fee for treatment, by procedure. *Preauthorization* indicates the insurance will or will not cover specific procedures as diagnosed by the dentist.

Both predetermination and preauthorization protect the dentist and the patient by informing them ahead of time exactly which procedures or treatments are covered by the insurer and the specific amount allowed (paid) by the insurance company. This helps eliminate confusion or misunderstandings after a procedure is started or completed and helps the patient understand his or her financial responsibility for the portion of treatment not covered by insurance.

Signature on File

Many dental insurers accept a **signature on file** status on all claims for the current *benefits year*. The office manager should check for the fiscal or policy year beginning and ending dates to ensure that the signature on file and the *Release and Assignment Forms* are updated, according to the requirements of the policy.

The *release* applies to dental records and authorizes the insurance claims examiners to review the diagnosis and treatment. Many procedures require dental radiographs to verify the need for treatment and the subsequent claim for payment.

The *assignment* refers to the benefit paid by the insurance company and authorizes the company to send payment directly to the dentist, rather than to the patient.

Most practices have a *"signature on file"* box on their new patient registration forms. When the patient first enrolls in the practice, he or she or the responsible party signs this box in lieu of having to sign an insurance claim form each time dental care is provided. The signature on file is also essential in practices that have electronic claims processing because there is no place to sign a form that is electronically submitted.

The final step in completing all the patient's forms is to file the insured patient's signature document. Most systems of claims submission now accept documentation that a current, legal signature is on file with the provider.

Walk-out Statement

At the conclusion of each treatment visit, many offices issue a **walk-out statement** to the patient or responsible party. The walk-out statement provides hand-written or computer-generated information including the patient's name, the date, the type of service provided, the insurance code, the fee, the amount paid, and the balance. The walk-out statement may be used by the responsible party in paying the statement personally, submitting the information to the employer's benefits administrator to receive direct reimbursement, or to personally submit to a third-party payor.

Use of Digital Radiographs and Intraoral Photographs

Most third-party carriers require preoperative (and occasionally postoperative) radiographs or intraoral photos supporting treatment submitted for payment. When insurance claims were submitted traditionally throughout the mail, radiographs or copies of original radiographs were often included in the envelope with the request for payment. This consumed the office manager's time, postage, and processing costs, and often delayed payment for six to eight weeks.

Today, most plans accept computer-generated images scanned and downloaded into their claims departments accompanying a computer-generated and transmitted statement. The average cost per computer-submitted claim is less than $1 and often takes only minutes to process. Another advantage to time and cost saving is supporting documentation cannot be lost in the mail, as is sometimes a problem with hard copy submissions.

The One-Write System

Although the majority of dental offices use computers for accounts receivable, some practices still use the *one-write* or *pegboard* manual system. The components of the system include a plastic or metal writing surface onto which prepunched, preprinted forms fit, using a system of raised pegs on the left side. Forms are designed to fit over each, using a carbonless transfer system. This eliminates the need to make duplicate bookkeeping entries, thus saving time and reducing mathematical errors.

The *daily journal sheet* or *day sheet* provides a listing of activities for each patient seen during the business day. Also, it serves as a method of recording payments received on account during the day.

The office manager manually enters the date, the patient's account number, the patient's name, and the service code. The office manager also enters in the necessary information under the columns designated for the fee charged, the payment received, the balance, and the previous balance.

The pegboard or one-write system also provides one-write *receipts, fee slips,* and *ledger cards,* onto which the information is automatically transferred using carbonless forms. The one-write ledger is stored in a *ledger file tray* and provides the office manager with an instant billing system. (A photocopy of the ledger becomes the patient's statement.)

Electronic Claims Processing

Electronic claims processing is one of the newest technologies available to assist dental practices in filing claims for payment. Electronic claims processing uses the practice's computer to store, generate, and submit third-party claims to respective insurance companies' computers via a clearinghouse.

Dental practices that utilize electronic claims processing find many advantages in this type of (paperless) claims submission:

- the predetermination cycle is almost always eliminated, saving valuable treatment time and paperwork;
- preoperative X-rays and study models are almost always unnecessary;
- saving on filing space, postage and paper processing costs (the average filing cost is $.75 to $1 per claim);

- quicker filing time;
- faster payment;
- security of direct deposit into the dentist's designated bank account (instead of processing and mailing paper checks); and
- fewer clerical errors.

Claims Tracking and Rejection

Occasionally, a claim may be lost, misplaced, or never received by the insurer. Whether using a manual or electronic method of claims processing, the wise office manager keeps a record of claims submitted by date, patient/responsible party's name, group number, insurer, and amount. If payment is not received within the customary timeframe anticipated, the office manager should contact the third-party to track the status of the claim.

Occasionally, a claim is rejected by the insurance carrier, most often because a vital piece of information has been omitted from the claim. This usually is the responsible party's social security number or group number. Missing codes or completed treatment records may also cause a claim to be rejected. A claim may be rejected because the insurance company does not cover the particular procedure. The office manager will note that in such cases, predetermination, and preauthorization would have caught this and it is her or his responsibility to make other financial arrangements with the patient before treatment commenced.

The wise office manager closely monitors the activity of all third-party claims. Therefore, it is essential that the business assistant keep a close watch on the payment activity of third-party claims. This is most efficiently conducted by printing out computer reports that supply a breakdown of payment on third-party receivables to obtain the following information:

- all claims that have been submitted for predetermination (if necessary)
- all outstanding claims submitted for payment
- charges for claims generated but not yet submitted
- claims that have been returned or rejected that have not been resubmitted

Methods of Payment

In addition to third-party payment, received either as paper checks or transferred electronically into the doctor's bank account, other methods of accepting payment for dental services are also utilized in the dental office. While monthly statements are most commonly used, the following forms of payment are used to collect receivables.

Cash and Cash Discounts

Cash is the preferred method of payment; as such, many practices offer a discount to cash-paying patients for prepayment of services in full. If the practice discounts for payment in full at the time of treatment, the full reduction applies to advance payment by cash or check. This way, patients who do not require statements save the practice the **costs of credit.** This saves the practice time and billing costs. The office manager must issue a receipt to the patient or responsible party for all cash sums paid.

Personal Check

Many patients prefer to pay their balance due by personal check. Paying by check has many advantages, including proof of payment through the canceled check; also, writing a check is safer than carrying large sums of cash.

Private Label Dental Care Cards

Contemporary issuers have created proprietary dental care cards, which offer credit lines up to $10,000 for qualified patients. One issuer is Healthcare® Creditline Dental (800-489-3279). "Loaded card" and "smart card" payment processing are becoming more commonplace. These programs involve prepayment or a similar program offered by the issuing institution, utilizing an embedded microchip to debit the card each time it is used against the prepaid amount.

The benefit to the office who participates is that payment is guaranteed and paperwork and processing time are reduced.

Credit Cards and Credit/Debit Card Readers

Acceptance of any type of credit card or granting credit in-house costs the practice a percentage of the fee. These options also carry a cost to the practice for accepting and processing most types of credit cards. Some issuers install the card reader for free; others assess a fee. The advantage of accepting major credit cards for payment is that payment is virtually guaranteed, and paperwork, billing, and collection time are reduced. Any finance charges are assumed by the patient.

If the practice accepts credit cards, the office manager displays the symbols and signage of the credit associations, such as VISA®, Master-Card®, American Express® and/or DiscoverCard®. This payment option should also appear on all statements sent out by the practice.

In some cases, patients do not have available limits on their personal credit cards to pay the remaining balance not covered by insurance preauthorization in a lump-sum. In these cases, the patient may agree to preauthorize the office manager to initiate a monthly charge to their credit cards in an amount and over an agreed upon timeframe necessary to make treatment affordable. While the credit card charges typically accrued by the practice are 2–6 percent, and it may take longer to receive payment in full, this amount is more than offset by the fact that no further collection or billing charges need be incurred.

Modern "point of sale" technology validates credit availability electronically, eliminating the risk of accepting an overlimit or expired credit card as payment; but this method of processing is not free. *Electronic credit account processors* are being compensated for this type of data access at a percentage of the fee. The cost is only a few cents on the dollar; however, processing fees should be considered before the decision is made to install the reader.

Direct Reimbursement

Direct reimbursement is a popular method of payment with dentists. The reason is that the patient may choose whomever he or she wishes as a provider of dental care. The patient pays the dentist's fee at the time of service and submits a copy of the paid receipt to his or her employer's benefits administrator. The administrator then generates a reimbursement check to the employee/patient, usually within 30 days.

Direct reimbursement plans usually have a ceiling amount of reimbursement per employee or per family per year or reimburse a percentage of the total fee. For example, the employer may cover 80 percent of all routine preventive treatments, 50 percent of all restorative treatment, and a flat, one-time benefit of $2,500 for orthodontic treatment.

In cases where the patient requires extensive dental treatment, the appointments may be planned in sequential phases throughout several benefits periods until treatment is completed. This maximizes the patient's return on direct reimbursement.

Series of Payments

Many patients prefer to take advantage of a series of payments (sometimes referred to as budget plans) to the doctor, especially if payment is made as treatment is being rendered. A series of payments is also amenable to the patient or responsible party if no interest charges are added to the total treatment.

Once the dentist has completed a diagnosis and treatment plan and the charges are explained to the patient with a copy of the treatment plan provided to the patient or responsible party in writing, it is the office manager's responsibility to make financial agreements.

An example of an agreement for a series of treatments is as follows. The total fee for Mr. Green's treatment is estimated at $1,800 and the treatment will take from three to six months to complete. Mr. Green states he would like to begin treatment and make monthly payments of $100 each for 18 months with no interest charges. The office manager explains that the doctor would like to be able to offer these terms to him; however, it is the doctor's policy that at least half of the treatment is paid for when treatment is initiated and payment-in-full by the final appointment.

The office manager then suggests to Mr. Green that he make a down payment of $1,000 at the initial appointment, with the additional sum of $200 due the 15th of each of the next four months, at which time the treatment will be completed. With Mr. Green's acceptance, the office manager completes a financial agreement statement, which is dated, signed by both parties, and so noted on Mr. Green's financial record (whether manually or by computer). One copy of the completed financial records goes into Mr. Green's file and another is given to Mr. Green. The office manager then sets up the necessary appointments for Mr. Green, being sure to allow sufficient time for lab work to be turned around between appointments. Note that if further time is required by Mr. Green to make payments or if finance charges are to be added, this information must be included in the financial agreement. Terms should also address the consequences should the patient not complete all planned treatment, fail to show for scheduled appointments, or fail to meet the terms of the agreement.

Cycle Billing

Cycle billing means statements (bills) are sent out on a regular, 30-day cycle. Some practices send out all statements on the same day of the month, and many indicate a due date to encourage patients to make payment promptly.

Other practices stagger the 30-day mail date of cycle billing, usually by dividing patients alphabetically by last names and billing a segment of the alphabet (A-D, E-K, L-P and Q-Z) each month. Staggering of statements makes processing easier in practices that send a large amount of statements to private-pay patients. This also evens out the cash flow throughout the month. While all practices vary somewhat in their receivables management, the following is an example of the typical life cycle of an account.

The Typical Billing/Collection Cycle

Cycle 1 – 30 days: The statement (bill) is mailed, usually at the end of the month, within 30 days or at completion of treatment.

Cycle 2 – 60 days: A second statement follows, usually with a sticker or other notation or a personally hand-written reminder from the office manager that payment is past due.

Cycle 3 – 75 days: At this time, the office manager should make the first formal telephone collection contact.

Cycle 4 – 90 days: If payment still has not been received, the office manager usually sends an ultimatum letter stating something to the effect of, "If payment is not received within 10 days, or if we have not heard from the financially responsible party in 10 days, this account will be turned over to a collection agency."

Finance Plans

Some practices prefer not to carry patients for any type of financing program and instead refer them to financing institutions such as local banks or programs sponsored in cooperation with the local dental association. Note that completion of a financial responsibility form is the office manager's responsibility when making initial records for all new patients (see *Chapter 10, Patient Records, Diagnosis and Treatment Planning* for further information.)

Under a financing program, the office manager may assist the patient or responsible party in completing a standard finance application and then fax or phone the information to the participating bank, credit union, or lending institution. Approval or denial is usually confirmed within 30 minutes.

If approved, the bank or lending institution provides payment in advance to the patient, made out in the dentist's name. The patient receives a coupon book that corresponds to monthly payments, similar to a mortgage or auto loan payment book. Fulfillment of the loan, including interest charges, is the responsibility of the patient or responsible party.

Procedure for Entering a Payment

Regardless of whether payment is made on a patient's account from a third-party, from the patient, or another financially responsible party, and whether using a manual, pegboard, or computerized accounts receivables system, the procedure for entering payments is the same.

If payment is made by check, the office manager endorses the check with the doctor's bank stamp. If payment is made in person by cash, the office manager provides the patient with an official receipt.

The office manager enters the amount of the payment on the patient's financial record, then the remaining amount due, if any. The payment is recorded on the bank deposit slip, which is totaled at the end of the day and deposited. Note that most dentists prefer to review the total accounts received for the day prior to making the bank deposit.

Performing a Credit Check

Many offices use credit checking services prior to beginning extensive cases. A credit check is legal, providing the patient is aware of the credit check and gives consent.

Credit checks may be performed using local credit agencies, either via telephone or electronically. The office is charged a fee for this service.

Collection of Past-due Accounts

It is most often the office manager's responsibility to collect overdue and/or delinquent accounts. The following general rules should be followed when collecting overdue balances.

Collection Telephone Calls

The office manager must follow certain rules or guidelines when making telephone collection calls. As such, the wise office manager makes every effort to communicate in a firm, business-like manner in a way that conveys, "Let's work together to resolve this issue." (She or he should never make threats, which only intimidate or alienate patients.) Following are general guidelines incorporated from the *Fair Debt and Collection Act*, which may be governed by laws that vary from state to state.

In general, the office manager should:

1. Make collection calls at a reasonable time (not before 8:00 a.m. or after 9:00 p.m.).
2. Identify herself/himself as collecting a debt only to the financially responsible party. She or he should not leave a message at the person's home or place of employment.
3. The office manager should identify himself or herself and the employer, as well as the nature of the call.
4. During a week, the office manager may only make a maximum of *two* calls to the delinquent party at his or her home; or a maximum of two calls to his or her place of employment during one month; a total of 10 calls is the maximum allowed. *Note:* Calls to the responsible party's workplace are *not* allowed if forbidden by the employer.
5. In placing collection calls, the office manager must keep in mind that she or he is a trained professional, and as such, may not harass, oppress, or abuse the financially responsible party. This behavior is not only unethical, but illegal, as well; it could possibly damage the professional reputation of the practice.

6. The office manager must not threaten further action if there is no intent of following through. Nor may she or he state that the patient's debt will influence his or her credit rating.

7. The office manager should thoroughly review the responsible party's account ledger or computer screen data and have specific amounts and dates readily available. If the responsible party makes specific statements about when he or she will pay and the amount, the office manager records this information. The office manager then summarizes what the responsible party agreed to.

8. Sometimes the amount of the balance or overdue debt is disputed by the patient. In this case, the office manger is prohibited from taking further action or contacting the debtor until sufficient verification can be provided. In this instance the office manager must send the responsible party written notice of his or her right to dispute the debt within five days of the initial communication. The responsible party then has 30 days from receipt of notification to take action. *Note:* Verification may be a copy of the statement of the overdue account or a copy of the agreement creating the debt.

9. If the responsible party sends the office a letter requesting that he or she not be contacted, the office must cease communication, except to notify the person of pending legal action.

10. *Note:* The office is entitled to incur interest and other charges to past due accounts only if the agreement creating the debt allows it or if it is permitted by individual state law.

Small Claims Court and Collection Agencies

If, after all traditional collection attempts are made and payment is still not received, the office has the final options of small claims court (civil court) or turning the account over to a collection agency, which will usually claim at least one-third of the moneys retrieved. Small claims court usually handles sums not in excess of $1,500. Before making such a drastic decision, always consult with the doctor as the final decision rests with him or her.

Skill-Building for Success: Student Activities

These optional activities and exercises are designed to help the student put into practice information learned in the chapter.

1. Your instructor will give you a sample insurance form to complete. Review the information required for completing an insurance form provided in the chapter. Using information provided by your instructor, complete the insurance form.

2. Mr. Alexander's account of $460 is 60 days past due and no payment has been received, despite having sent two statements. You bring this to the attention of the dentist, who instructs you to place a collection call to Mr. Alexander. Divide into pairs and take turns role-playing the office manager and Mr. Alexander. Be persistent. Do not back down. Ask probing questions of Mr. Alexander. Invite feedback and coaching strategies from your classmates. Have you stayed within the collection guidelines provided?

3. Mrs. Garcia calls the office and is very angry. She tells you that she has paid her account in full but just received a bill, which does not reflect her final payment. Divide into pairs and role-play the scenario. Ask your classmates for feedback. How could this scenario have been prevented? What steps should have been taken?

Skills Mastery Assessment: Post-Test

Directions: Select the response that *best* answers each of the following questions. Only one response is correct.

1. Advantages to the dentist of signing onto a managed care program include:

   a. a guaranteed flow of new patients
   b. minimal administrative costs
   c. a guaranteed cash flow and patient base
   d. all of the above

2. In a *group model* HMO the HMO contracts with an individual provider group to care for its patients. The provider group is managed independently and reimbursed on a capitated basis.

   a. True
   b. False

3. In an EPO plan, all dental services provided by unaffiliated providers are automatically reimbursed.

   a. True
   b. False

4. Claims are rejected by the insurance carrier due to all of the following common reasons *except:*

   a. missing responsible party's social security number or group number
   b. missing codes or completed treatment records
   c. the patient had a change of address
   d. procedures are not covered by the carrier

5. All of the following are true of PPO providers *except:*

   a. they are selected based upon their professional qualifications and performance
   b. they benefit through decreased patient volume
   c. they must agree to a fee schedule and review of their performance
   d. they receive prompt payment for services rendered to patients enrolled in the plan

6. The term third-party means someone other than the dentist or the patient is involved in financial responsibility for treatment.
   a. True
   b. False

7. Information required for claims submission for payment includes:
   a. the name of the insured party, the responsible party, the spouse, or parent or guardian of the insured party
   b. the name of the employer, employer code, or group number
   c. the address and telephone number for submitting claims and the acceptable method(s) for claims submission(s)
   d. all of the above may be required

8. The term *deductible* refers to:
   a. the amount the insurance company pays toward services covered under the contractual plan
   b. the company that sells or carries the insurance
   c. the amount the patient or responsible party must pay toward services before the carrier will begin paying on insurance claims
   d. the extent of the insurance policy (e.g., the benefits included)

9. Treatment codes are necessary when filing for third-party reimbursement to:
   a. ensure that each procedure is properly billed
   b. ensure that the correct amount is paid to the provider
   c. ensure dual coverage benefits
   d. a and b only

10. Predetermination indicates whether the insurance will or will not cover specific procedures diagnosed by the dentist as necessary.
    a. True
    b. False

11. Procedures for which no code is provided are generally reimbursed when the patient has proof of insurance coverage.
    a. True
    b. False

12. The term *release* applies to dental records and authorizes the insurance claims examiners to review the diagnosis and treatment. Many procedures require dental radiographs to verify the need for treatment and the subsequent claim for payment.
   a. True
   b. False

13. The term *assignment* refers to the benefit paid by the insurance company and authorizes the company to send payment directly to the patient, rather than to the provider.
   a. True
   b. False

14. The walk-out statement provides hand-written or computer-generated information including all of the following *except:*
   a. the patient's name and the date
   b. the patient's date of birth
   c. the type of service provided
   d. the insurance code, the fee, the amount paid, and the balance, if any

15. The walk-out statement may be used by the financially responsible party to:
   a. pay the statement personally
   b. submit the information to his or her employer's benefits administrator to receive direct reimbursement
   c. personally submit to a third-party payor
   d. all of the above

16. Electronic claims processing uses the practice's computer to store, generate, and submit third-party claims to respective insurance companies' computers via a clearinghouse.
   a. True
   b. False

17. Advantages of electronic (paperless) claims processing may include:
   a. elimination of the predetermination cycle, which saves valuable treatment time and paperwork
   b. saving on filing space, postage, and paper processing costs
   c. The security of direct deposit into the dentist's designated bank account
   d. all of the above

18. Reasons for rejection of payment on a claim by the insurance carrier may include any or all of the following *except:*
    a. missing codes or completed treatment records
    b. missing the responsible party's social security number or group number
    c. missing the patient's middle name
    d. the insurance company does not cover the particular procedure

19. The office manager should issue a receipt to the patient or responsible party for all cash sums paid.
    a. True
    b. False

20. According to the guidelines set forth by the *Fair Debt and Collection Act,* the office manager should:
    a. identify herself or himself as collecting a debt only to the financially responsible party
    b. not leave a message at the person's home or place of employment
    c. not make calls to the responsible party's workplace if *not* allowed or forbidden by the employer
    d. all of the above

References

Blair/McGill Advisory. (1995, December).

Dietz, E. (1997). *Career enrichment: Expand the skills you have to create the job you want.* Falls Church, VA: National Association of Dental Assistants.

Dietz, E. (1996). *Office management for the busy dental assistant: How to balance a career with professionalism.* Falls Church, VA: National Association of Dental Assistants.

Direct reimbursement: Tailor your own employee dental benefit plan. Chicago, IL: Author.

Domer (1996, Spring). Managed care, associateship and practice purchase. *Preview.*

Finkbeiner B. (1995). *Practice management for the dental team* (4th ed.). St. Louis: Mosby.

Glossary of managed care terms. (1996, March). *ACCESS.* Chicago, IL: ADHA.

Position paper on managed care. (1996). Chicago: American Dental Hygienists' Association.

The ultimate computer system illustration guide. (1990). Phoenix, AZ: Practice Outlook®, Inc.

Torres, H., Erhlich, A., Bird, D., & Dietz, E. (1995). *Modern dental assisting* (5th ed.). Philadelphia: W.B. Saunders.

Chapter 13

Managing Accounts Payable

- **Understanding Accounts Payable**
  When an Invoice Arrives
  Embezzlement
- **Understanding Overhead**
  Fixed Expenses
  Variable Expenses
- **Controlling Practice Overhead Through Budget Goals**
  Categories of Practice Expenses
- **The Office Checking Account**
  Components of a Check
  Bank Deposits
- **Understanding the Bank Statement**
  Reconciling the Bank Statement
- **Electronic Funds Transfer and Automatic Payments Systems**
- **Other Forms of Payment**
  Petty Cash
  Cash on Delivery (COD)
  Charge Cards
- **Payroll Records and Reporting Procedures**
  Employer Identification Number
  Employee's Withholding Allowance Certificate
  Employee Earnings Record
  Payroll Deductions
  Depositing Withheld Income Tax and Social Security (FICA) Taxes
  Federal Unemployment Tax
  Wage and Tax Statement
  Report of Withheld Income Tax
  Retaining Payroll and Tax Records

Learning Objectives

Upon completion of this chapter, the student will achieve an 80 percent or higher score on the Skills Mastery Assessment Post-Test *covering the following material.*

1. Define the term overhead as it pertains to the dental practice.
2. Define and differentiate between fixed and variable overhead expenses associated with the dental practice.
3. Be familiar with the most commonly used forms of accounts payable, including check writing systems, electronic wiring of funds, and other computerized payment systems used by the office manager; also the seriousness and consequences of embezzlement.
4. Be familiar with common categories of overhead and types of expenditures associated with dental practice including handling COD payments, automatic deposits, and monthly expenditures.
5. Describe standard taxes withheld from employee paychecks and the importance of sound record keeping for all payroll procedures.
6. Describe and list the purposes of common tax forms and required payments, including quarterly filing and annual employee withholding statements.

Key Terms

accounts payable	fixed expenses
automatic payment systems	overhead
cash on delivery (COD)	petty cash voucher
electronic funds transfer	restrictive endorsement
embezzlement	variable expenses

Understanding Accounts Payable

Chapter 12 addressed accounts receivable in the office. This chapter addresses **accounts payable,** the system of distributing money owed by the practice. It is the office manager's job to ensure that the accounts payable duties are conducted efficiently, accurately, honestly, ethically, and in a timely manner.

Often, the office manager is responsible for the distribution of large sums of money owed by the practice to a variety of suppliers, government tax agencies, and other vendors. Accurate accounting methods are essential to maintain an efficient system of bookkeeping, including accounts payable.

The office manager may be expected to perform the following tasks associated with maintaining receivables: writing checks, endorsing checks and making bank (or electronic) deposits, keeping accurate account balances, and reconciling bank statements.

When an Invoice Arrives

When an invoice (bill or statement) arrives, the office manager should check the vendor's invoice number against the original packing slip or the invoice enclosed to ensure they are for the same amount and that all goods or services ordered were indeed delivered. Invoices should be filed alphabetically by vendor, paid monthly, and retained for three years.

Embezzlement

The wise office manager realizes she or he has responsibility for ensuring that all bookkeeping functions of the practice balance, as she or he may be held accountable for any discrepancies. Further, the claim of **embezzlement** (the fraudulent appropriation of money entrusted into one's care) is a serious allegation that if proven, may result in immediate termination, denial of unemployment benefits, failure to find future employment, and possible indictment, imprisonment, and/or fines.

Understanding Overhead

The term **overhead** means the operating expenses associated with running the dental practice. Expenses included in overhead include such items as the rent or mortgage payment; property taxes (if applicable); payroll and independent contractor expenses; outside consultants, including legal and accounting services; supplies, dental laboratory bills, utility bills (electricity, heat, water, garbage removal), parking; marketing costs; insurance premiums; other services not included with payroll such as cleaning and housekeeping, laundry and dry cleaning; outdoor maintenance such as landscaping, tree-trimming, and snow removal; continuing education, professional association fees; equipment warranty/service contracts; front office and stationery supplies; professional and waiting area publications; entertainment; professional licensing, incorporation fees, and more.

When faced with such an enormous list of overhead expenses, the office manager may feel overwhelmed at keeping them organized, let alone paid in a timely manner. In most dental practices today, the average overhead runs at 70 percent or higher.

Fixed Expenses

The term **fixed expenses** includes those office expenses which remain fairly constant from month to month. These are generally the larger bills, such as rent or mortgage, payroll, utilities, and lease payments on equipment.

Variable Expenses

The term **variable expenses** includes those office expenses which vary from month to month, or are received only on occasion. These may include dental supplies and lab fees, new equipment purchases, and new services.

Controlling Practice Overhead
Through Budget Goals

Many dental practices set annual budgeting goals as a cost-containment strategy. Just as they establish production goals to achieve maximum practice revenues, budget goals help contain costs incurred by the practice. Some practices reward the office manager by keeping practice overhead revenues within an established percentage of production.

Categories of Practice Expenses

The following categories and percentages of practice overhead may be used as a guide in determining anticipated office expenses at annual budget review time. They are based upon gross collections of a solo practitioner office.

Personnel Expenses

The highest overhead associated with personnel is payroll, including salaries and taxes, which average between 18 percent and 25 percent. Another 2 percent to 4 percent of personnel benefits goes toward employee benefits.

Occupancy Expenses

The cost of physical occupancy of the practice may run from 5 percent to 9 percent. This includes the lease note plus interest, depreciation, insurance on the building and contents, janitorial and maintenance services, and some utilities.

Administrative Expenses

The cost of administering the practice may run 6 percent to 9 percent and includes accounting and legal services, collection costs, and bank charges, related computer expenses, continuing education, dues and subscriptions, insurance (including disability, malpractice and business overhead), laundry and dry cleaning, licenses and permits, front office and printing supplies, postage, repairs and maintenance to equipment, taxes, telephone, and other miscellaneous administrative expenses.

Equipment and Furnishings

The cost of equipment and furnishings may run 4 percent to 6 percent and includes lease notes and interest on equipment and/or cash purchases of equipment. This cost may be as high as 25 percent in new practices.

Clinical/Dental Supplies

The cost of dental supplies associated with patient care may run from 4 percent to 7 percent. However, the incurment of additional infection control and barrier protection costs associated with compliance with government regulations may raise this cost to 10 percent to 12 percent.

Lab Fees

The cost of dental lab fees varies greatly, depending upon the type of practice and volume of prosthetic or orthodontic cases. Generally, lab fees range from 2 percent to 4 percent.

Marketing Costs

The cost for marketing expenses also varies from practice to practice. Marketing costs may include giveaways, gifts and donations, telephone directory space advertisements, practice newsletters, holiday cards, mailings, and media costs. Experts currently establish marketing costs at 5 percent of the practice's overhead budget.

The Office Checking Account

The office checking account is the primary means by which bills (accounts payable) are paid. Most bills are paid on a monthly basis. Payroll is paid weekly, biweekly, bimonthly, or monthly. In most practices, only the dentist/owner of the practice has the authority to sign checks. In some offices two signatures are required as a system of checks and balances for checks to be payable. These signatures may be of the dentist/owner and the office manager or some other major share-holder of the practice. Some practices grant power of attorney to the office manager to sign checks. The signature of the person authorized to sign checks must be on file with the bank where the account is held.

It is the office manager's duty to ensure that all bills and payroll are paid promptly and correctly. Ensuring that bills are paid on time establishes a good credit rating for the practice and eliminates additional interest or carrying (finance) charges assessed for late payment. This saves the practice money in the long-term.

Regardless of whether the office uses a manual check writing system, a one-write check writing system, or a computerized software check writing system, the following components of check writing apply.

Components of a Check

A check is a written order to the dentist's bank to pay a specified amount of money to a designated person *(payee)*. Writing a check requires entering or displaying the following minimal information.

The *Magnetic Ink Character Recognition (MICR)* numbers are encoded along the bottom of the check to facilitate high-speed machine processing. The first part of this number is the bank's ABA (American Bankers Association) identification number; the second part is the maker's (dentist's) checking account number. The name of the bank also appears on the check. Each check is individually sequentially numbered at the top of the check for easy tracking.

The name and related information about the *payor* (the dentist or representative of the practice) is printed at the top of the check, usually at the left side, usually including the practice's address. The date the check is written must be filled in, as well as the name of the *payee* (the person or organization to whom the funds are payable, for example, "*ABC Dental Supply, Inc.*").

The amount of the check must be entered two different ways. This is required to reduce the incidence of error and for clarification by the bank, should a question arise about the exact amount. The *numerical amount* of the check is entered first, such as *$233.86.* It is then entered in long hand, typed, or keystroked into the computer as *"Two hundred thirty-three and _____ 86/100"* on the next line. Note the long dash or wavy line following *and,* which is used to prevent alteration of the original amount for which the check was written.

Many checks also feature a *memo line* for the payee to make note of the reason or purpose for writing the check, for example, *dental supplies.* Finally, the payor's signature line is where the payor signs at the bottom (Figure 13-1).

Note that it is imperative that this identical information be recorded in the checkbook stub area, which corresponds to the number of the check written. The wise office manager completes the check stub portion (sometimes referred to as the check tracker) first, to avoid confusion as to the amount of the check, the date written, or the name of the party to whom the check was written. This saves embarrassment, confusion, and valuable time later.

When making out a check for an especially large amount of funds, the office manager may elect to make a photocopy of the check, should it be required at some time in the future as proof of payment.

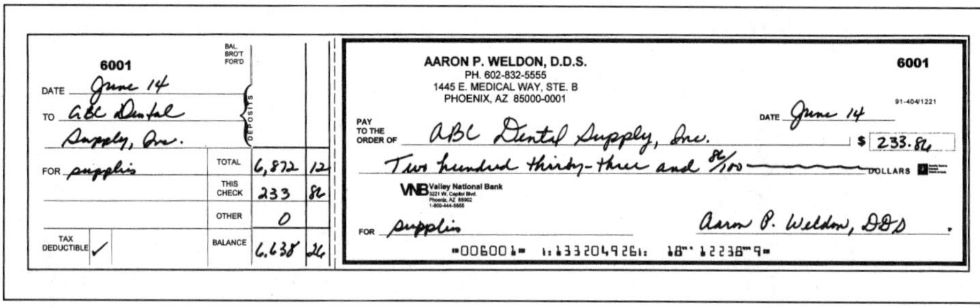
6001
DATE June 14
TO ABC Dental Supply, Inc.
FOR supplies
TAX DEDUCTIBLE ✓
BAL. BRO'T FOR'D
DEPOSITS
TOTAL 6,872 12
THIS CHECK 233 86
OTHER 0
BALANCE 6,638 26
AARON P. WELDON, D.D.S.
PH. 602-832-5555
1445 E. MEDICAL WAY, STE. B
PHOENIX, AZ 85000-0001
6001
DATE June 14
PAY TO THE ORDER OF ABC Dental Supply, Inc.
$ 233.86
Two hundred thirty-three and 86/100 DOLLARS
Valley National Bank
FOR supplies
Aaron P. Weldon, DDS

Figure 13-1. Sample check.

Bank Deposits

Another important role in maintaining the practice's checking account is preparing the nightly deposit for the bank. Most often it is the responsibility of the office manager to prepare the daily *bank deposit slip* in preparation for deposit. In some practices, the office manager is also personally responsible for making the deposit. In other practices, the dentist completes this task. Note that deposits may be made in person at the bank, by mail, by night deposit, or at an *automatic teller machine (ATM).*

When the dentist opens a checking account, *deposit slips* are printed with the dentist's or practice's name and account number. Spaces are provided to enter the date and the totaled amounts of checks and cash to be deposited. Whether using the manual check deposit system, a one-write system, or a computer software banking program, the process for making bank deposits is the same.

Prior to depositing checks into the account, each check must be endorsed by the *payee* (the dentist/practice to whom the check is written). Endorsement may be made by signing the back of the check or using an ink-stamp **restrictive endorsement.** Note that if the check is signed, for example, *"Dr. Ralph Jones,"* anyone finding that check may attempt to redeem it for cash at a bank. *This is called a blank or open endorsement and is not recommended for security purposes.*

The restrictive endorsement contains special conditions or restrictions limiting the receiver of the check concerning use that can be made of the check. Most often the ink-stamp endorsement reads, *"For Deposit Only"* on the first line and features the doctor's name or the name of the practice on the second line—*"Ralph Jones, DDS."* This significantly reduces the potential for bank fraud.

When making a manual deposit, the office manager lists the name of each patient next to the amount of the check. When making cash deposits, the office manager makes a list of patients and the corresponding amount paid and clips it to the duplicate deposit slip.

The deposit slip is made out manually or computer generated from the day sheet. Note that creating a computer-generated deposit slip from the day sheet significantly reduces the likelihood of a error, omission, or embezzlement, as it provides a detailed account sheet of *all* patients scheduled for the day including those for whom no charge or payment was entered or received.

Many offices make a photocopy of each production day's deposit slip as a method of tracking daily deposit amounts.

Understanding the Bank Statement

The bank provides a monthly bank statement containing all checks (by chronological number) cleared and all deposits made by amount and date the transaction occurred. Other items that appear on a monthly bank statement may include overdrafts, interest accrued, bank service and ATM charges, printed check charges and electronic payments such as federal withholding tax, as well as the starting, ending balances (Figure 13-2).

The office manager should promptly review the bank statement upon receipt carefully, to ensure that no errors have occurred (banks *do* make mistakes) and that all deposits were duly noted. The office manager should then *reconcile* the bank statement. Note that some banks return the physical checks, while others retain them on *microfiche* and send only the bank statement. Because not all checks written on the office account are cleared (cashed) immediately, it is necessary to reconcile the statement to determine the exact amount in the account.

Reconciling the Bank Statement

To maintain an accurate checking account record and statement balance, the office manager is responsible for reconciling the bank statement. The following steps are necessary:

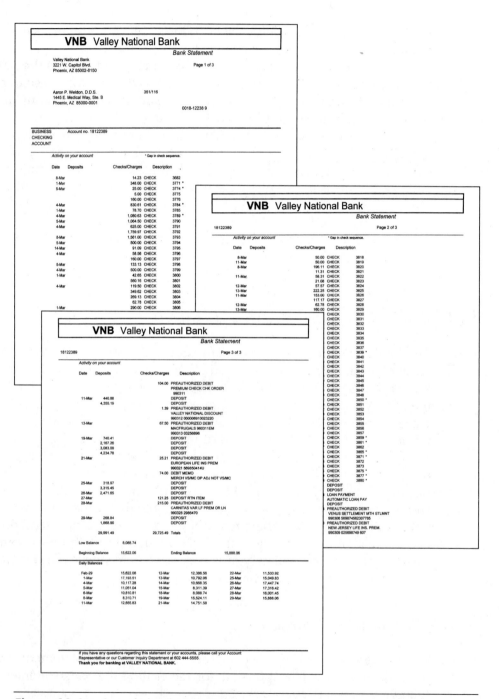

Figure 13-2. Sample bank statement.

1. Compare and verify the amount of the canceled checks with the amounts indicated on the bank statement. The office manager will note that the canceled checks, or the check numbers printed on the statement, will be arranged or reported sequentially.

2. Arrange the canceled checks in chronological order (if enclosed with the statement).

3. Compare the amounts reported on the canceled checks and the deposits to the amounts entered into the checkbook register at the time the check and deposits were made. Indicate with a check mark or other visual symbol all canceled checks and deposits in the checkbook register.

4. List any *outstanding checks* (those not returned to the bank for payment) with the corresponding check number and the amount of each. Total the amounts of the outstanding checks.

5. If a deposit was made but does not appear anywhere on the bank statement, add the amount to the bank statement balance. Likewise, if the account is *interest earning*, add that amount. Subtract and total the amount of the outstanding checks.

6. Review other charges listed on the bank statement such as service charges, debit memos, ATM privilege charges, automatic withdrawals or overdrafts, and subtract them from the checkbook register.

Bank statements and canceled checks (if returned from the bank) should be retained for seven years, in case they are required for an audit.

Electronic Funds Transfer and Automatic Payments Systems

Some practices prefer to save time by using **electronic funds transfer** and/ or **automatic payment systems** to pay routine bills.

Electronic transfer of funds may be conducted over the telephone by relaying specific information to a bank representative to move funds from one account to another. The bank or financial institution representative informs the caller that the conversation is being recorded and requests personal identification information to ensure the validity of the request. This helps prevent the likelihood of fraud or other funds transfer that could result in costly overdraft charges.

Automatic payment systems automatically deduct the amount of a specific payment, for example a utility payment, automobile payment, a newspaper subscription, or a charge card balance from the payor's checking account every month by prearrangement and deposit the amount to the account of the party owed. This saves time, paper, and postage costs of writing and mailing a check.

Other Forms of Payment

While check-writing is the preferred type of payment system used by dental practices in accounts receivable management, other forms of payment are also used, including petty cash, **cash on delivery (COD)**, and charge cards.

Petty Cash

While the office manager is strongly advised against storing large sums of money in the office, out-of-pocket expenses sometimes arise. Occasionally, a small amount of cash is needed to make change for a cash-paying patient or for lunches, tips for delivery personnel, etc. (Note that petty cash generally rarely exceeds $50.)

When such expenditures are required, often on short notice, the office manager is responsible for completing a **petty cash voucher** as a receipt of proof of outlay of cash. Preprinted petty cash vouchers or forms may be purchased from a stationery supply company, or, the office may elect to create a hand-written petty cash voucher for minimal expenses.

Information contained on the petty cash voucher should include the date, the person or party to whom the cash was paid, the reason for the payment, and the name or initials of the person who distributed the monies.

Cash on Delivery (COD)

Occasionally, supplies or vendors require payment at the time of delivery, rather than through a monthly billing procedure. This is called cash on delivery, abbreviated COD. Such a delivery may be paid for from the petty cash fund.

Occasionally, COD orders exceed $50 and many vendors will accept (or prefer) a check upon delivery. In this instance the office manager may draft a check for the total and obtain the doctor's signature at the time of delivery. Before doing so, however, she or he should check the contents of the package against the packing slip to ensure the goods are intact and are what was ordered.

Charge Cards

Occasionally the practice may make purchases using charge cards, especially while away from the practice attending continuing education seminars, for airline tickets, hotel accommodations, and meals. When a charge card is used for payment, the office manager must keep a file of charge card receipts, the reason for the expenditure, and the amount due. This amount is compared with the monthly charge card statement for accuracy.

At the direction of the dentist, the office manager writes a check for the entire amount due, a portion of the amount due, or the minimum amount due. Note that late payment or partial payment on a charge account accrues interest charges.

Payroll Records and Reporting Procedures

Depending upon the size of the staff and amount of the payroll, some practices prefer to handle payroll in-house, either manually or electronically on a computer soft-ware system; others prefer to have an outside payroll administration company administer payroll.

Whether preparing the payroll information for in-house administration or for an outside agency, it is most often the office manager's responsibility to maintain accurate payroll records and other accounting procedures.

Federal and state laws require records to be kept on information regarding wages paid and for the preparation of required tax reports. The dentist/employer must obtain a copy of the Internal Revenue Service's *Employer's Tax Guide-Circular E,* which summarizes the employer's responsibility for computing, depositing, paying, and reporting all taxes. The office manager should be aware that laws change frequently and that a current copy of this table should be kept on file for the latest withholding and reporting information.

Employer Identification Number

As an employer, the dentist must have an *employer identification number*. This is a nine-digit number assigned to either sole proprietors or corporations for the purpose of filing and reporting payroll information as required by the federal government. This may be applied for through the Internal Revenue Service as *Form SS-4*.

Employee's Withholding Allowance Certificate

Each employee of the practice must complete an *Employee's Withholding Allowance Certificate, Form W-4*. The withholding certificate determines the status of each staff member for income tax deductions from earned wages. The following information is required on this form: the employee's full name, Social Security Number (SSN), home address, marital status, total number of allowances (exemptions) claimed, and any additional amount desired to be withheld. The employee must sign and date the form. If the employee changes the number of exemptions claimed (dependents), a new *Form W-4* must be completed.

Employee Earnings Record

By law, the dentist as employer must maintain all employees' earnings records, including a summary of individual staff member's earnings. This information is important because it provides the employer with information required for quarterly and annual tax reporting. Although varying somewhat, the employee's earnings record should provide the following general information:

1. The employee's name, address, Social Security Number, rate of pay (hourly or salaried), the number of withholding exemptions claimed, marital status, and any other special deductions, including garnishments for child support, automatic savings programs, or health insurance or retirement plan contributions.
2. The number of pay periods in a reporting quarter and the date when each pay period ends.
3. Regular earnings, overtime earnings, and total earnings.
4. A column for each type of deduction and total deductions.

5. The net amount paid to the employee or *net pay*. (Net refers to the amount paid after deductions are taken from the *gross pay*.)

6. Accumulated taxable earnings, which gives the employer information for taxable earnings, FICA, and taxable wages for contributions to unemployment taxes.

7. Amounts for quarterly and annual totals. This information is used when the employer submits quarterly and annual tax payments and reports.

Payroll Deductions

At the time of employment, a specific wage is determined by the employer. This may be hourly or a salaried amount set weekly, biweekly, bimonthly, or monthly. Often, the office manager is responsible for calculating deductions and determining net wages reflected in paychecks.

Note: Confidentiality regarding payroll is a must! The office manager may not discuss payroll with any other staff members as this constitutes a breach of confidentiality and may be grounds for dismissal!

FICA: Federal Insurance Contributions Act (Social Security and Medicare Taxes)

These deduction amounts vary from year to year and differ with the amount of income earned. It is the dentist/employer's responsibility to seek out the latest information in payroll tax deductions.

The Social Security portion is a flat percentage based upon the first $60,000 earned. The Medicare tax is a flat percentage on all earnings with no ceiling amount.

Tax tables are available free of charge from the Internal Revenue Service. *An Employer's Tax Guide—Circular E* with a sliding scale can be obtained from the IRS and used for easy reference.

Withholding (Income Tax Deductions)

The amount of withholding tax varies depending upon the number of exemptions the employee claims on the employee's *W-4 Form*. The more exemptions claimed, the less tax withheld. Thus, two employees earning the same amount may have differing net or take-home pay, depending upon the number of exemptions claimed and marital status.

Local income tax may be deducted by some cities and states that have personal income taxes. Other withholding amounts may include automatic savings to a bank or credit union, child support, etc.

After computing the individual employee's net pay, checks are written or the information is sent to a payroll processing company outside the office who will use the initial information submitted and automatically print out checks.

The information is then recorded on each staff member's individual earning record. If a one-write or pegboard accounting system is used, the information on the employee's earnings is recorded directly onto the earnings record, as well as the monthly expense disbursement sheets when the check stubs are recorded. This reduces the amount of time required and also helps eliminate human computing errors.

Depositing Withheld Income Tax and Social Security (FICA) Taxes

The Internal Revenue Service automatically sends the dentist/employer a Federal Tax Deposit (FTD) Coupon Book *(Form 8109)* with coupons to deposit all types of taxes. Additional forms can be obtained or ordered using the *FTD Reorder Form (Form 8109A)*.

For clarification, the dentist/employer owes taxes when the wages are paid, not when the payroll period ends. Instructions provided in completing *Form 941* provide further information. Returns and tax payments are due as follows. *Note:* It is now possible to do this by telephone for the IRS to make electronic tranfer.

Quarter	Quarter Ends	Date Pmt. Due
#1: January–March	March 31	April 30
#2: April–June	June 30	July 31
#3: July–September	September 30	October 31
#4: October–December	December 31	January 31

Federal Unemployment Tax

The employer/dentist must also pay federal unemployment tax on each employee at the rate of 6.2 percent of the first $7,000 in earned income. Note that employees do not contribute to unemployment benefits funds— only employers do.

The dentist must determine federal unemployment taxes quarterly and deposit the amount on or before the last date of the first month after the close of the corresponding quarter, reporting with *Form 941* on or before January 31st.

Wage and Tax Statement

Each year the dentist/employer must supply for each employee a copy of *Form W-2, Wage and Tax Statement*, no later than January 31st. This information is crucial because the employee must supply this when filing his or her personal income tax return (for both state and federal agencies).

A total of six copies of the *W-2 Form* are provided. One copy is for the Internal Revenue Service, one for the state, city or local tax department, three copies to the employee (one for federal tax return filing, one for state or local tax filing, and one for the employee's permanent files); a final copy is retained by the dentist/employer.

The *W-2 Wage and Tax Statement Form* contains the following important information:

1. The Employer's Identification Number, name, and address
2. The employee's Social Security Number, name, and address
3. The amount of federal income tax withheld
4. The total sum of wages paid the employee
5. The total FICA employee tax withheld
6. The total wages paid subject to FICA
7. All state and local taxes withheld, where applicable

Report of Withheld Income Tax

The dentist/employer must also submit, on or before February 28th of each year, copy A of all *W-2 Forms* issued for the previous year and *Form W-3, Transmittal of Wage and Tax Statements*, to the IRS.

Retaining Payroll and Tax Records

It is the responsibility of the dentist/employer to retain all records regarding employment taxes, for at least four years following the date of taxes they pertain to, should the IRS order an *audit.* The following information is the minimum that should be retained by the employer regarding employee payroll and tax records:

1. The amounts and dates of all wages paid to employees
2. The names, addresses, occupations, and Social Security Numbers of all employees
3. The dates of all staff members' employment
4. Any periods in which employees were paid while absent due to illness or occupational injury
5. All employees' income tax withholding allowance certificates
6. The employer's identification number
7. Copies of returns filed with dates and amounts of required deposits made

Skill-Building for Success: Student Activities

These optional activities and exercises are designed to help the student put into practice information learned in the chapter.

1. Contact the IRS for a copy of *An Employer's Tax Guide—Circular E.* Using the charts provided by the IRS, determine the net pay for a dental assistant earning $600 per week, who is married and claims two exemptions.
2. Invite a payroll administration company representative to visit your class to provide a demonstration of how payroll is administered outside a small business, such as a dental office.
3. Bring in a copy of your personal checking account monthly statement. Using the steps provided in the chapter, reconcile your checking account.
4. Using the percentages for specific types of budgeting of office overhead provided in the chapter, set up a hypothetical budget for a practice having a $300,000 production budget. (*Note:* approximately 30 percent should be applied to the dentist's income.) Compare your figures to those of your classmates.

Skills Mastery Assessment: Post-Test

Directions: Select the response that *best* answers each of the following questions. Only one response is correct.

1. Accounts payable is a system of/for:
   a. distributing money owed by the practice
   b. collecting money owed to the practice
   c. making collection calls to patients who have overdue bills with the practice
   d. receiving direct reimbursement from insurance companies

2. Which of the following procedures may the office manager be expected to perform related to managing accounts receivable?
   a. writing checks
   b. making bank deposits
   c. reconciling bank statements
   d. all of the above

3. The term overhead pertains to the operating expenses associated with running the dental practice.
   a. True
   b. False

4. _____ overhead includes those office expenses which remain fairly constant from month to month.
   a. variable
   b. income
   c. fixed
   d. reconciled

5. Embezzlement is a serious charge that may result in:
   a. immediate termination
   b. denial of unemployment benefits
   c. possible arrest, imprisonment, and/or fines
   d. any or all of the above

6. In many dental practices today the average overhead runs at _____ percent or higher.

   a. 50
   b. 60
   c. 70
   d. 90

7. The cost of administering the practice includes all of the following *except:*

   a. accounting and legal services
   b. collection costs and bank charges
   c. payroll
   d. continuing education, dues, and subscriptions

8. The signature of the person authorized to sign checks must be on file with the bank where the account is held.

   a. True
   b. False

9. Ensuring that bills are paid on time:

   a. establishes a good credit rating for the practice
   b. eliminates additional interest or carrying (finance) charges assessed for late payment
   c. saves the practice money
   d. all of the above

10. The *Magnetic Ink Character Recognition (MICR)* numbers are encoded along the bottom of a check:

   a. facilitate high-speed machine processing
   b. include the bank's ABA (American Bankers Association) identification number
   c. include the customer's checking account number
   d. all of the above

11. When writing a check, the office manager should complete the check stub portion after completely filling out the check.

   a. True
   b. False

12. A/an _____ endorsement contains special conditions or restrictions limiting the receiver of the check concerning use that can be made of the check.
    a. blank or open
    b. closed
    c. restricted
    d. implied

13. The monthly bank statement lists:
    a. all checks (by chronological number) cleared and all deposits made by amount and date the transaction occurred
    b. overdrafts, interest accrued, and bank service charges
    c. starting and ending balances
    d. all of the above

14. When reconciling the office checking account the office manager should:
    a. list any outstanding checks with the corresponding check number and the amount of each
    b. total the amounts of the outstanding checks
    c. indicate with a check mark or other visual symbol all canceled checks and deposits in the checkbook register
    d. all of the above

15. Automatic payment systems automatically deduct the amount of a specific payment from the payor's checking account every month by prearrangement and deposit the amount to the account of the party owed.
    a. True
    b. False

16. A petty cash voucher is a receipt of proof of outlay of cash.
    a. True
    b. False

17. The employer identification number:

    a. is a nine-digit number assigned to either sole proprietors or corporations for the purpose of filing and reporting payroll information as required by the federal government

    b. may be applied for through the Internal Revenue Service as Form SS-4

    c. replaces the dentist's Social Security Number (SSN)

    d. a and b only

18. An *Employee's Withholding Allowance Certificate, Form W-4:*

    a. remains the same throughout the duration of employment

    b. requires the employee's full name, Social Security Number (SSN), home address, marital status, total number of allowances (exemptions) claimed, and any additional amount desired to be withheld

    c. determines the status of each staff member for income tax deductions from earned wages

    d. b and c, only

19. The employee's earnings record provides the following information:

    a. the employee's name, address, Social Security Number, rate of pay, the number of withholding exemptions claimed, marital status and any other special deductions, including garnishments for child support, automatic savings programs or health insurance or retirement plan contributions

    b. the number of pay periods in a reporting quarter, the date when each pay period ended, regular earnings, overtime earnings, and total earnings

    c. the total deductions, the net amount paid to the employee, accumulated taxable earnings, amounts for quarterly and annual totals for the employer to use when submitting quarterly, and annual tax payments and reports

    d. all of the above

20. The *W-2 Wage and Tax Statement Form* contains the following *except:*

    a. the Employer's Identification Number, name, and address

    b. the total sum of wages paid the employee

    c. the employee's spouse's Social Security Number

    d. the total FICA employee tax withheld

References

Dickey, K. W. (1995, Spring). Understanding overhead. *Preview.*

Finkbeiner, B. L., & Allan, C. (1995). *Practice management for the dental team* (4th ed.). St. Louis: Mosby.

Griffin, A. P. Categories of expenses based on gross collections [Handout].

Griffin, A. P. *Analysis of current activities in the practice.* Greenville, NC: Practicon, Inc.

Chapter 14

Supply Ordering and Inventory Control

- **The Importance of Managing Supply Inventory**
- **Types of Supplies**
  Consumable Supplies
  Disposable Supplies
  Expendable Supplies
  Equipment
- **Managing Supply Quantity Needs of the Practice**
  Shelf Life
  Rotating Stock
  Storage Considerations
  Rate of Use, Reorder Point, and Flagging System
  Storage of Controlled Substances
- **Computerized Ordering and Inventory Control**
- **Quantity Discounts**
  Buying in Bulk
  Automatic Shipments
  Bids and Contract Buying
- **Supply Order Tracking**
  Order Form
  Purchase Order
  Packing Slip
  Invoice
  Backorder
  Credit Invoice
- **Warranties and Repairs**

Learning Objectives

Upon completion of this chapter, the student will achieve an 80 percent or higher score on the Skills Mastery Assessment Post-Test *covering the following material.*

1. Describe the office manager's role in managing dental office supply inventory.
2. Describe the necessary steps in tracking and managing supply quantity needs of the office.
3. Define supply inventory terms, such as shelf life, rotating stock, and storage considerations.
4. Describe the necessity of security precautions for in-office drug inventory and dispensing.
5. List the steps (manual or electronic) in supply ordering and inventory control.
6. Be familiar with the methods of saving the office money on supplies, including bulk quantity purchases, automatic shipments, and contract purchases.
7. Understand the terms associated with dental supply ordering and receipt, such as packing slip, back order, and credit invoice.
8. Describe the office manager's role in maintaining equipment warranties and service repairs.

Key Terms

automatic shipments	flagging system
backorder	inventory
consumable supplies	invoice
credit invoice	packing slip
disposable supplies	purchase order
expendable supplies	purchase order number
equipment	quantity discounts

Key Terms (cont.)

rate of use

reorder point

shelf life

supplier/vendor

warranty

The Importance of Managing Supply Inventory

An important part of the office manager's job is maintaining a sufficient amount of dental supply items and purchasing them at the lowest price. Because most dental practices spend upward of 10 percent of their total overhead on dental supplies, the supply budget represents a significant expenditure by the office and must be managed accordingly.

Types of Supplies

Supplies may be broken down into four categories: **consumable, disposable, expendable,** and **equipment.**

Consumable Supplies

Consumable supplies are those that are completely used up or consumed with use. These include anticariogenic agents, cements, impression materials, and gypsum products.

Disposable Supplies

Disposables are single-use items that are discarded immediately after the procedure for which they are used. These include paper cups, exam gloves, dental dam, cotton rolls, anesthetic needles, and carpules.

Expendable Supplies

Expendable supplies are those items that are relatively low in cost and are replaced frequently. These include paper clips, burs, matrix bands, and plastic impression trays.

Equipment

Equipment items are those major purchases that are used for five or more years and may be depreciated by the office over a number of years. These include such items as computers, chairs, dental units, sterilizers, lasers, handpieces, and intraoral cameras.

Managing Supply Quantity Needs of the Practice

In purchasing and reordering supplies it is important to note that a sufficient quantity must be ordered so as not to run out of a necessary item, while taking care not to order too many units only to have insufficient storage space or to determine that the **shelf life** may expire before the item can be used.

Shelf Life

The shelf life is the amount of time a product is guaranteed fresh. The product should be used before it reaches the expiration date marked on the label and discarded after the expiration date. Examples of items with a shelf life include prescription medications, cements, impression materials, and dental X-ray film (Figure 14-1).

Rotating Stock

The office manager must ensure that when new supply items are received in the office the oldest items are used first; new items are placed farthest back in the storage area and brought forward as the older items are removed from the front. This ensures product freshness; also to keep products and supplies from becoming "lost" in storage.

To ensure an organized supply storage area, the office manager should label shelves, cupboards and bins appropriately with the product name or type of product for easy retrieval. Examples include, *"patient bibs,"* *"cements,"* *"HVE tips,"* *"burs,"* *"alginate,"* *"dental dam,"* *"restorative materials,"* etc.

Guidelines for Storing Supplies

Following are helpful suggestions for the office manager in storing supplies:

- **Store supplies in one central area.** Keeping them together helps make maintenance and inventory easy.
- **Keep a minimum amount of product on hand.** Maintaining too many supplies costs the practice money and many products have a shelf life.
- **Be alert to products that are light- or heat-sensitive.** Read all bottles and package labels to check for expiration dates and storage instructions. This includes items such as gloves, cements, and anesthetics.
- **Use storage bins to organize supplies.** Plastic or cardboard bins that are high in back and low in front help facilitate rotation and avoid expiration of shelf life. They also keep hard-to-stack items neat and organized.
- **Plan to spend a minimum of one hour each week to check supplies, determine reorder points, and throw away outdated supplies.**

(Adapted from Taking stock: How to order, store and maintain dental supplies, by Jill L. Sherer.)

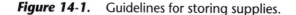

Figure 14-1.   Guidelines for storing supplies.

Storage Considerations

Consideration must be given to special storage requirements on product labels, such as light and heat sensitivity (i.e., refrigeration, storing in a cool dark area or keeping certain hazardous materials apart from each other). For example, as referenced in *Chapter 2, Legal and Ethical Issues and Responsibilities,* ammonia and bleach should not be stored next to each other, as they may cause an explosion; also, the resulting fumes may be fatal, if inhaled.

Note items for use in the operatory that require special storage. For example, dental film must be stored at not less than 50° nor more than 70°, but not under refrigeration due to excess moisture build-up. Items that do require refrigeration must be stored separately from edible items, such as staff lunches and beverages.

Rate of Use, Reorder Point, and Flagging System

Offices vary widely in the quantity of supplies used and the rate at which they use them. Many office managers determine a **rate of use** on commonly used items to establish a routine **reorder point** for each. Rate of use refers to the rate of consumption of items and supplies commonly used in the office. The reorder point is a predetermined minimum quantity of a specific supply left in inventory. When the item reaches the minimum quantity, additional units are to be ordered to avoid running out, especially if the item is backordered by the supplier.

If using a manual system for supply inventory and reordering, a **flagging system** may be used to signal the predetermined reorder point. If a computerized system is used, the computer will automatically alert the office manager to the appropriate reorder time when the item is taken out of inventory at the reorder point.

Storage of Controlled Substances

Today, more offices stock and dispense controlled (narcotic) or other prescription drugs as a convenience to patients. To prevent abuse of controlled substances, unauthorized dispersement or theft, the office that dispenses these prescription medications should use a *double-lock storage system*.

A double-lock system requires two separate keys to open the storage box. Two different people in the office must each maintain one key, independent of the other.

Dispensing of prescription drugs also requires that known drug allergies and sensitivities be entered into the computer data base for each patient, as well as other known medications taken by the patient. This is to prevent the likelihood of overdosing or double-dosing patients, as well as dispensing two or more drugs that may cause an adverse reaction or serious side effect (*drug synergism*) if taken simultaneously by the patient.

Computerized Ordering and Inventory Control

Many practices take advantage of computerized supply ordering and inventory control. Having the capability to order supplies by computer also facilitates printing out a list of supplies by name, manufacturer, usage rate, and reorder time required.

The office manager may use a computer wand across the bar code on the product label or package at reorder time, or may use specific software provided by the individual **supplier/vendor** (company from whom the office orders supplies.) The advantages of ordering supplies via the computer electronically are *time savings* in order processing and receipt and *avoidance of duplication* of orders.

Quantity Discounts

Because offices spend a significant amount of money on supplies annually, they often take advantage of suppliers' **quantity discounts.** Quantity discounts are extended to offices for buying large numbers or units of a single item to receive a discount per unit. This is also called *buying in bulk.*

Buying in Bulk

In an effort to save the office money on supplier special and large order quantity discounts, the office manager may be tempted to order excessive amounts of products. Careful planning must take into consideration the *rate* at which consumables, disposables, and expendables are used, the *amount* of available storage space, and the need for *special storage.*

For example, a case of cotton rolls normally sells for $29.95 and the quantity discount rate is three cases at $26.95 each, or 12 cases for $23.95 each. The office would save $3 per case by buying three (a $9 saving) or it would save $6 per case by buying 12 cases (a $72 saving).

If the office has sufficient space to store 12 cases of cotton rolls and uses them quickly, this may represent a significant saving to the doctor. Because cotton rolls require no special storage requirements (such as refrigeration), the cost saving may be justified. If, however, few cotton rolls are used, or storage space is minimal, it may be wiser to order a smaller amount.

Automatic Shipments

Many offices take advantage of quantity discounts or bulk purchases and save valuable storage space at the same time. When storage considerations, product freshness, or rate of use are of concern, they may still take advantage of these savings through **automatic shipments** arranged with an individual supplier.

For example, if an office uses two cases of gloves monthly (24 per year), the office manager may wish to take advantage of a supplier's special on gloves (at the quantity discount rate), but may not have enough space to store large quantities of cases of gloves. Using an automatic shipment plan, the office manager may order the gloves at the lowest price per case (based on 24 cases per year) and arrange with the supplier to have two cases shipped automatically on the same day each month. The office benefits by always having a fresh supply of gloves available, without bulky storage requirements.

Bids and Contract Buying

Many large group offices and clinics prefer to send their supply needs out on *bid* and enter into an annual *contract* with the supplier who bids the lowest on the total supply budget for the year.

This system is helpful in relying on one supplier for the majority of dental supplies purchased for the year and helps the office maintain a sound **inventory** supply system. The inventory is a written or computer-printed list that includes all supplies on hand, the amount ordered, the manufacturer/supplier, the reorder frequency (approximately how often to place another order), and the per unit price.

Supply Order Tracking

Part of the office manager's job is to order supplies and track all paperwork and records for accuracy and to ensure proper payment for invoices.

Order Form

An initial order for a product or supply is placed through a vendor, manufacturer, or supplier. This may be in person with a dental supply sales representative, a manufacturer's representative, over the telephone, by fax, by mail, or via the computer (including e-mail and websites). Regardless of how the order is placed, a uniform set of information is necessary to complete the order.

Information necessary to place an order includes the name of the vendor/supplier, the appropriate address, telephone or fax number, the quantity, the item number, a description of the product, and any other important information, such as size, shade, unit pricing, etc.

The vendor/supplier will need to know from the office manager the doctor's name and full mailing address, telephone number, and account number. If there are special shipping considerations, such as days the practice is open to receive a package, or that an item is to be held until a specific date, the vendor/supplier will also need to know this information (Figure 14-2).

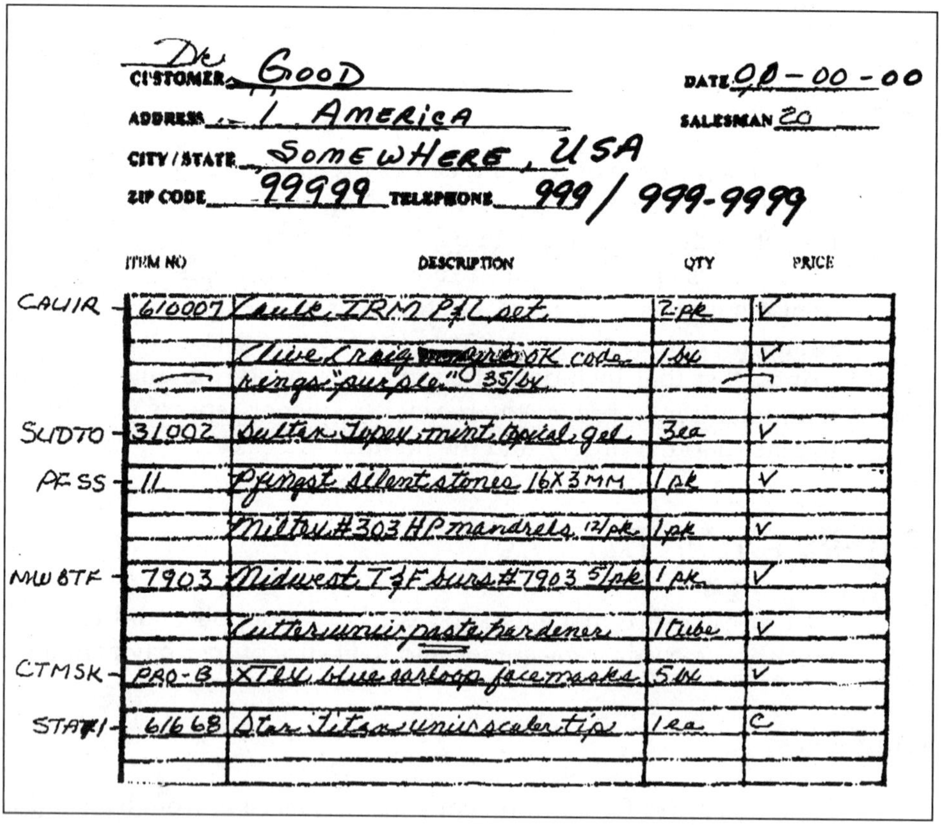

CUSTOMER Dr. GOOD DATE 00-00-00
ADDRESS 1 AMERICA SALESMAN 20
CITY/STATE SOMEWHERE, USA
ZIP CODE 99999 TELEPHONE 999/999-9999

	ITEM NO	DESCRIPTION	QTY	PRICE
CAUIR	610007	Caulk IRM P/L set	2 pk	✓
		Clive Craig OK code rings "purple" 35/bx	1 bx	✓
SUDTO	31002	Sultan Topex mint topical gel	3 ea	✓
PF SS	11	Pfingst silent stones 16X3MM	1 pk	✓
		Miltex #303 HP mandrels 12/pk	1 pk	✓
MW 8TF	7903	Midwest T&F burs #7903 5/pk	1 pk	✓
		Cutters univ paste hardener	1 tube	✓
CTMSK	PRO-B	XTRA blue earloop facemasks	5 bx	✓
STAR1	61668	Star Titan univ scaler tip	1 ea	C

Figure 14-2. Sample order form. *(reprinted courtesy Valley Dental Supply Inc., Burbank, CA.)*

Purchase Order

Large practices and clinics sometimes place their orders, either on paper or electronically, using a **purchase order.** A purchase order contains the practice, clinic or institution's name, customer number, and all other pertinent order information.

An additional significant piece of information required on every purchase order is a **purchase order number.** The purchase order appears, usually using a sequentially ordered numbering system, in the same location on each purchase order. When placing an initial order or referring to an existing purchase or repair requisition, the purchase order number is vital. It should be used on all correspondence and communications with a vendor.

Packing Slip

After the order has been placed, the merchandise will arrive at the office. It is the office manager's duty to sign for the packages received if delivered by a vendor and to review the contents of the package for accuracy.

Inside the package or outer envelope is a **packing slip**, which lists the contents of the package. This information should be identical to the order form and the subsequent invoice, which is a bill requesting payment for merchandise. The office manager should review the information contained on the packing slip and compare it to the original order and the final invoice for payment. She or he should note any errors, omissions, discontinued items, or backordered items. If there are discrepancies, she or he should contact the vendor immediately.

Invoice

After the order has been received and marked off against the original order, the items must be put away in the appropriate storage areas of the office. Within 30 days the office will receive an **invoice** requesting payment for the items sent.

The office manager must once again check the items and prices listed on the original order against the packing slip and the invoice to ensure accuracy of billing. The invoice will note a date of payment due (Figure 14-3).

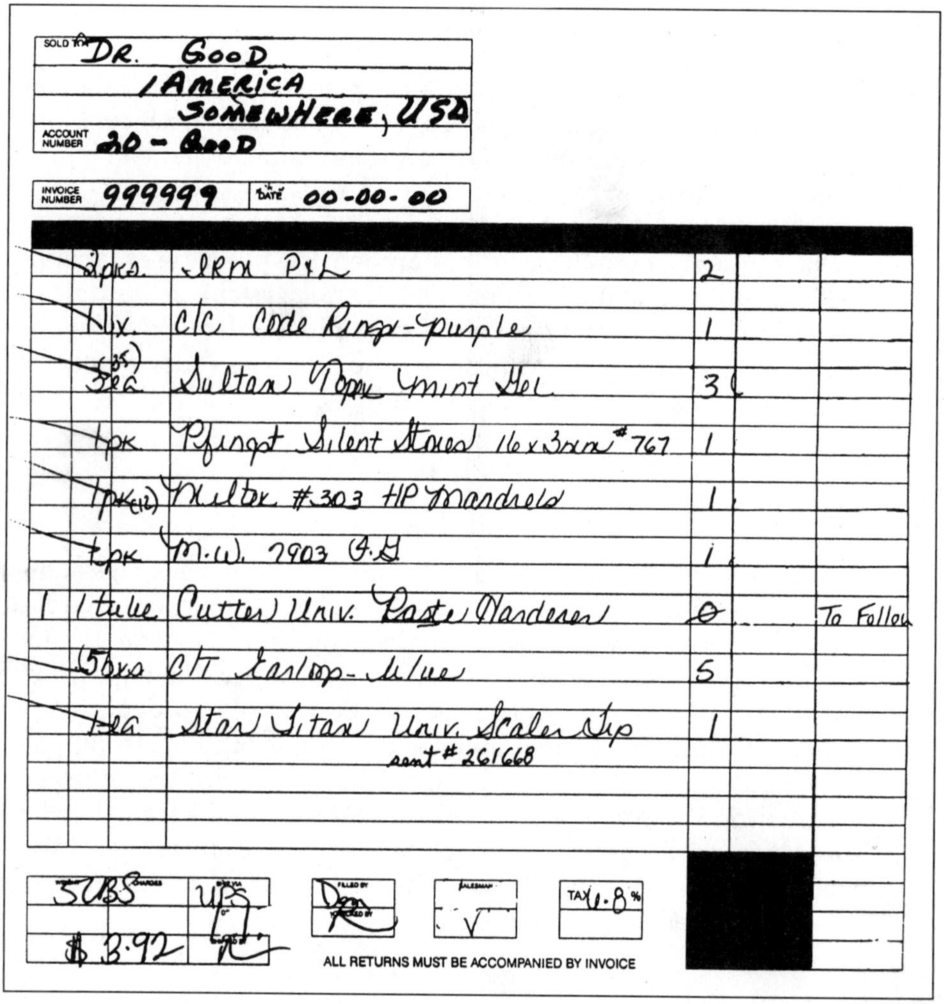

Figure 14-3.   Sample invoice. *(reprinted courtesy Valley Dental Supply Inc., Burbank, CA.)*

Backorder

Occasionally, items ordered are not in stock with the vendor/supplier and are not shipped with the other items on the original order. In this instance, the item is placed on **backorder.** This means that when the vendor/

supplier receives the product it will be shipped separately to the dentist's office as part of the original order.

The office manager should take care to not place a duplicate order when checking on a backordered item, and likewise, that the office is not charged twice for one order (Figure 14-4).

Credit Invoice

Occasionally, the office will cancel an order or return an item for a refund. In this instance, the vendor/supplier may issue a **credit invoice** for the items canceled or returned.

A credit invoice works exactly opposite of an invoice (statement) and may be deducted from the bill or may be credited to the dentist's account toward a future purchase.

Warranties and Repairs

Part of the job of maintaining control of inventory is that of overseeing repairs and warranties on purchases and equipment of the practice.

Occasionally, a service representative must be contacted to repair existing equipment or install replacement parts. Similar to invoices for supplies, equipment repairs must also be tracked for accuracy.

Warranties on large pieces of equipment should be filed or stored in a designated place in the office for easy access and reference. In instances where equipment has outstanding warranty on repair or parts, this information must be readily accessible when arranging for repairs or replacement.

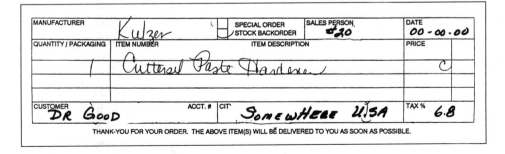

Figure 14-4. Sample backorder slip. *(reprinted courtesy Valley Dental Supply Inc., Burbank, CA.)*

Skill-Building for Success: Student Activities

These optional activities and exercises are designed to help the student put into practice information learned in the chapter.

1. The dentist has asked you to place an order for one case of Caulk fast-set alginate, one bottle of Durelon™ Cement and three #11R Buffalo Dental spatulas from ABC Dental Supply. Using the information provided, role-play placing a telephone order for the items requested; and make up the doctor's name, address, and telephone number. The office will be closed for vacation next week and you would like the items delivered after Tuesday, the 20th of the month.

2. Break into small groups or teams to solve the following problem. A salesperson calls or stops in at your office with an excellent buy on personalized toothbrushes (only $.35 each). The offer is good only for today and you must order 5,000 units to take advantage of this special offer. The doctor is out of the office attending a continuing education seminar in another state. The office is running low on toothbrushes. What should you do? (Estimated discussion time: five to 10 minutes.) Following discussion in your group or team, share your resolution and your rationale with the class.

3. You open an order from XYZ Dental Supply only to find that you have been billed twice for one item and that two other items are missing; however you were billed for them. What should you do?

Skills Mastery Assessment: Post-Test

Directions: Select the response that *best* answers each of the following questions. Only one response is correct.

1. Which of the following is *not* an important part of the office manager's job in inventory control and management:
   a. maintaining a sufficient amount of dental supplies
   b. purchasing supplies at the lowest price
   c. depleting inventory to the last unit before reordering
   d. working with suppliers

2. Consumable supplies are single-use items that are discarded immediately after the procedure for which they are used.
   a. True
   b. False

3. Because most dental practices spend upward of 10 percent of their total overhead on dental supplies, the supply budget represents an insignificant expenditure.
   a. True
   b. False

4. Which of the following is *not* considered an equipment item?
   a. plants in the reception area supplied and maintained by an outside florist
   b. an intraoral camera
   c. items that may be depreciated by the office over a number of years
   d. major purchases that are used for five or more years

5. If the shelf life of a product has expired, the office manager should:
   a. tell the chairside assistant to use it anyway
   b. discard the item
   c. call the supplier for an exchange or refund
   d. place the item on backorder

6. In maintaining and storing supplies, the office manager should:
   a. store supplies in one central area
   b. spend a minimum of one hour each week to check supplies, determine reorder points and throw away outdated supplies
   c. be alert to products that are light or heat sensitive
   d. all of the above

7. To ensure product freshness, the office manager should arrange supplies with the newest farthest back on the shelf and the oldest brought forward to be used first.
   a. True
   b. False

8. Special storage considerations for products the office manager must consider include:
   a. storage requirement information on product labels
   b. heat sensitivity
   c. light sensitivity
   d. all of the above

9. A double-lock storage system:
   a. prevents abuse of controlled substances
   b. controls unauthorized dispersement or theft
   c. requires two separate keys held by two different people to open the storage box
   d. all of the above

10. Supplies for use in the operatory that require refrigeration may be stored in the same refrigerator with items for personal consumption, such as lunches and beverages.
    a. True
    b. False

11. Which of the following is a benefit of entering an order via the computer?
    a. time saving in order processing and receipt time
    b. increased order accuracy
    c. automatic shipment
    d. guaranteed lowest pricing

12. With careful planning, the office manager may save the practice money on the supply budget using:
    a. bulk purchasing
    b. automatic shipments
    c. annual purchasing contracts
    d. all of the above

13. The packing slip:
    a. lists the contents of the package
    b. should be identical to the original order form and to the subsequent invoice
    c. notes backordered items
    d. all of the above

14. A backorder means that when the supplier receives the product it will be shipped separately to the dentist's office as part of the original order.
    a. True
    b. False

15. If the office manager notices a discrepancy on the packing slip he or she should:
    a. refuse to accept the delivery for partial shipment
    b. wait until the order is completed before checking off the contents
    c. contact the supplier immediately
    d. place an order for the missing items with another supplier

16. A credit invoice may be deducted from the bill or may be credited to the dentist's account toward a future purchase.
    a. True
    b. False

17. The office manager should keep a separate file of equipment warranties in the event of a repair or replacement problem.
    a. True
    b. False

18. The supply inventory is a written or computer-printed list that contains:
    a. all supplies on hand
    b. the usual amount ordered
    c. the manufacturer/supplier
    d. all of the above

19. A case of patient bibs normally sells for $24.95. The office manager has the opportunity to save money by ordering 12 cases at $21.45 per case. If he or she places the order for 12 cases at the quantity discount rate, how much will the practice save on this order?
    a. $2.50 per case, for a total saving of $30
    b. $3.50 per case, for a total saving of $42
    c. $4.50 per case, for a total saving of $54
    d. $5.00 per case, for a total saving of $60

20. Careful planning of supply ordering and inventory control must take into consideration:
    a. the rate at which consumables, disposables, and expendables are used
    b. the amount of available storage space in the office
    c. special storage requirements
    d. all of the above

References

Cost-cutting tips you can use. (1996, August). *Journal of the American Dental Assistants Association, Vol 127*.

Engel, P. New options in dental supply purchasing. *Progressive Dentistry*.

Proper drug dispensing and storage reduces risks. (1997, November/December). *Dental Insurance and Claims News, SAFECO Vol 12,* 6.

Sherer, J. (1992, October). Taking stock: How to order, store and maintain dental supplies. *AGD Impact: Business Watch*.

Smith, C. Dispensing more than advice: A growing number of dentists look at dispensing medications from their offices. *Progressive Dentistry*.

Vasquez, B. (1997, Winter). Everyone wins!! Systems, communication needed for successful dental office-lab relationship. *Dental Equipment and Supplies* [insert]. *Dental Economics*.

Chapter 15

Employment Opportunities

- **Type of Employment Desired**
  - Solo Practice
  - Group Practice
  - Managed Care Facility
  - Specialty Practice
- **Employment Opportunity Sources**
  - Newspapers
  - Dental Associations
  - Electronic Sources: The Internet, E-Mail, and Websites
  - Campus Placement Programs
  - Telephone Directories
  - Dental Supply Sales Representatives
  - Employment Agencies
  - Employee Leasing Organizations
- **Preparing for Employment**
  - Preparing a Résumé
  - Preparing a Cover Letter
- **Preparing for the Interview**
  - Appropriate Dress and Professional Demeanor
  - Plan Ahead
  - During the Interview
  - Information That May Not Be Discussed
  - Authorization to Release References and Other Information
  - Drug Testing
  - After the Interview
- **Terms of Employment**
  - Letter of Employment
  - Provisional Employment
  - Salary Negotiations

- **Other Career Opportunities in Dentistry**
  Teaching
  Sales: Retail Supply Houses, Dental Manufacturers,
      and Telemarketing Organizations
  Dental Consultant
  Dental School Clinics
  Government Clinics, Public Health, and Correctional Facilities
  State Board of Dental Examiners
  Insurance/Managed Care Corporate Offices

Learning Objectives

Upon completion of this chapter, the student will achieve an 80 percent or higher score on the Skills Mastery Assessment Post-Test *covering the following material.*

1. Describe the types of practices where the office manager might seek employment.
2. List employment opportunity sources.
3. Describe the steps in preparing for employment.
4. Describe the steps in preparing for an interview.
5. Be familiar with terms relating to employment.
6. Describe other dental employment opportunities outside of traditional private practice.

Key Terms

cover letter   reference
group practice   résumé
interview   solo practice
managed care

Whether starting out in his or her career, reentering the job market after family transition or as an experienced team member, the office manager must search out a number of employment opportunities for the best possible job. The wise office manager plans a strategy to access as many leads as possible.

Type of Employment Desired

At one time, a vast number of dental office manager positions were in fee-for-service private, **solo practices.** Today, there are numerous options for employment, including the following. The wise office manager will examine a number of opportunities prior to accepting a position.

Solo Practice

Today, about two-thirds of all dental practices are privately owned by one dentist, offering fee-for-service procedures. The trend is fast changing, however, due to a variety of factors including the increase in group practices to share overhead expenses, the increase in managed care practices, and the growing number of specialty practices.

Group Practice

The **group practice** (an office owned or operated by two or more dentists or other share-holders) may represent a greater challenge for the office manager who enjoys a busy environment and who may enjoy the responsibility of scheduling, supervising, and conducting performance appraisals of other staff members.

The rise in group practices is due to increasing overhead costs (including the cost of complying with government regulations and infection-control requirements) and decreasing revenues for procedures paid by third-party payors (insurance companies and managed care corporations).

Managed Care Facility

Many **managed care facilities** operate identically to privately owned practices; however, the dentists and other providers of care (hygienists) may be on contract with one or several managed care companies. The office manager may find it helpful to fully analyze the nature of employment, as well as the compensation and other benefits provided by managed care corporations prior to accepting a position.

Specialty Practice

The specialty practice provides a unique opportunity to serve dental patients requiring a narrower, more specialized field of dental treatment (see *Chapter 1, Introduction to the Dental Team* for a complete listing and description of the eight recognized dental specialties).

Employment Opportunity Sources

The wise office manager contacts a variety of sources of employment. Consideration must be given not only to the *type of practice*, but also the *geographic location* and commuting distance. Following are a variety of employment sources.

Newspapers

Classified sections of Sunday newspapers represent the greatest selection of employment opportunities. Generally located under "healthcare," opportunities are listed alphabetically as "dental assistant," "dental office manager," etc. Occasionally, specialty practices will appear alphabetically farther down the healthcare column (for example, as "orthodontic assistant").

Many classified advertisements are run as *blind ads*, which means the identity of the employer is not disclosed to the applicant. This is to ensure confidentiality of the employer/dentist. It also reduces the number of telephone inquiries that may flood the office the day after the advertisement appears.

Some classified advertisements require candidates to mail, fax, or e-mail a résumé to a Post Office Box, office, or home fax machine or to an e-mail site electronically. Again, this is to ensure confidentiality of the employer.

Dental Associations

Some state dental associations have an employment referral service to match their dentist-members with potential employment candidates. Of the states who provide this service, many offer it at no cost as a benefit to their members.

The office manager moving from out of state may wish to consider the city or geographic area of desired employment and to have this information available when contacting the dental association.

Electronic Sources: The Internet, E-Mail, and Websites

Many larger employers now offer the employment option of sending a résumé or job inquiry via the computer over the *Internet*. This may be done by sending to an *e-mail* address obtained from a *website*. The advantages of job searching through electronic sources to the employment candidate are speed of inquiry and savings on postage and paper. The advantage to the employer is the ability to scan résumés into a database for instant retrieval.

Campus Placement Programs

Most post-secondary campuses have a placement office that posts ongoing job openings for students and alumni (graduates) of their programs. This service is offered free of charge and is frequently updated. The goal of campus placement programs is to match students with employers in the area.

Telephone Directories

When sourcing employment in large metropolitan areas, the office manager may wish to consult telephone directories and Yellow Pages listings for dental employment opportunities in specific suburbs or areas within the city.

Dental Supply Sales Representatives

Dental supply sales representatives cover a specific geographic or regional area (territory) and are often aware of open dental office positions within their sales territories. The office manager may contact local dental supply houses to speak with sales representatives who cover territories within their desired area of employment.

Employment Agencies

Employment agencies are privately owned or franchised companies who prescreen and pretest applicants for employers. They work on a flat fee or commission basis to place ads, prescreen applicants, and conduct preliminary employment interviews before sending applicants to interview with the prospective dentist/employer.

Some dentists prefer to work through employment agencies, paying a percentage based on the salary paid to the candidate selected to save screening time and administrative costs.

Employee Leasing Organizations

Many employers, especially owners of large clinics, find it efficient to lease employees, rather than hire them outright. This saves the employer (and office manager) a significant time investing in advertising, screening, interviewing, and hiring. It is also useful in finding replacements to cover vacations and maternity and sick leave.

Leasing companies also handle payroll, administration of benefits, and other human resources services for the dentist.

Preparing for Employment

Once the geographic area and types of employment desired have been determined, it is time to prepare for employment. This includes developing a **résumé** (or multiple résumés), a **cover letter,** getting ready for actual interviews, and being prepared for follow-up.

Preparing a Résumé

A résumé is a review of the candidate's credentials that states his or her qualifications for employment. It contains the candidate's biographical information (name, address, and current telephone number), the type of employment sought, and education and previous work experience pertinent to desired employment.

There are two types of résumés: *chronological* and *functional*. A chronological résumé states the job objective, the work history in reverse order (most recent first), education, personal characteristics, and resources. A functional résumé states skills and experience related to the job. This is used by career reentry candidates or where the candidate has held a variety of jobs and wishes to focus on one area of employment.

Preparing a solid résumé is crucial to getting a good job. Following are résumé rules adapted from Robert Half, Founder of Robert Half International, Inc.

- Always print your résumé on standard letter size, white or ivory rag paper. (Avoid excessively bright colors or other distractors.)
- Always print out your résumé with plenty of space between paragraphs or sections and allow for adequate margins. Note that many large organizations use *scanners,* which are computerized machines with OCR (optical character recognition) that pick up specific key words. Thus, the office manager should use the exact word or words in describing the type of job sought (for example, "dental assistant," "dental office manager," etc.).
- Avoid use of fancy or excessive type styles, charts, or graphics in a résumé. Standard fonts such as Helvetica, Geneva, Arial, Times Roman, and Courier (American Typewriter) work well.
- Always use conventional English and good grammar. Avoid polysyllabic words, slang, and excessive verbs.
- Use short paragraphs or sections. Using too many words makes it difficult for the reviewer to absorb all information; stick to main points and key phrases.
- Always have someone else proofread your résumé.
- Always develop the résumé geared toward a specific job. This takes additional work, but with a computer or word processor, multiple versions of a résumé can be stored. For example, if the advertisement is for a dental office manager of a large orthodontic practice, the employment desired should reflect that: "Orthodontic practice manager."
- If you have had previous employment, always include specific contributions or improvements made in that position. For example, "Increased collections by 16 percent in 12 months."
- Give greater emphasis to previous employment that has greater relevance to the job you are currently seeking. For example, if you worked as a waitress between semesters, you may list this as college employment; however, focus on the desired position, "office manager."

- Always list affiliations or membership in professional or civic associations, where appropriate. If, for example, you volunteered at an oral health fair or are a member of the ADAA, list these items.
- Always keep a permanent file of your professional achievements. This is not only a good basis for your résumé, it is also essential in seeking a raise or promotion.
- Always reread your résumé just before an interview—chances are the interviewer just did that too!
- Always tell the truth.

Likewise, there is certain information that should *not* be included in preparing a résumé:

- Never give reasons for termination or leaving a job on a résumé.
- Never take more than two lines to list hobbies, sports, or other personal or social activities.
- Never include your **references** (names of people who could provide a job recommendation), Social Security number, spouse's occupation, or personal philosophies on the résumé.
- Avoid using exact dates of employment or education; months and years are sufficient. If you were out of the workforce for a number of years, you may wish to prepare a functional résumé, rather than a dated one.
- Never include your present employer's telephone number unless your boss is aware of your eminent departure.
- Avoid using professional jargon, unless dental terminology that will be understood by the person interviewing you.
- Never include salary information on a résumé. You may actually shortchange your earning power in doing so (Figure 15-1) (Figure 15-2)!

Preparing a Cover Letter

A résumé, alone, is an insufficient response to a classified advertisement or other notification of an opening. Although the well-prepared résumé may accurately reflect all work experience, credentials, and the desired position, an explanation of the intent must accompany the initial inquiry.

Sandra Wolfe, CDA
2664 N. Deans Mill Way
Saratoga, NY 12973

POSITION DESIRED: **Dental Office Manager**

WORK EXPERIENCE: **Office Manager/Receptionist** – Dr. David Rubin

Responsible for all incoming and outgoing calls;
computer scheduling and statement generation;
responsible for all third-party claims filing, including electronic claims processing.

June 1998 – present

Chairside Assistant – Dr. George Watkins

Performed all chairside functions, including four-
handed dentistry, OSHA compliance for infection
control and hazard communication; ordered all
supplies; X-ray certified.

December 1995 – May 1998

EDUCATION: **Niagara County Community College Dental
Assisting Program** – 1994 graduate

Saratoga High School – 1993 graduate

RELATED QUALIFICATIONS AND ACTIVITIES:

CPR Certified (American Red Cross)

CDA, CDPMA – Dental Assisting National Board

Volunteer – Tri-Cities Oral Health Fair

Figure 15-1. Sample chronological résumé.

This explanation is a cover letter, and must accompany the original
résumé, whether mailed, faxed, or e-mailed, in response to a job inquiry. A
cover letter introduces the candidate and explains the reason for the

Sandra Wolfe, CDA
2664 N. Deans Mill Way
Saratoga, NY 12973

POSITION DESIRED: Office Manager in a Group Dental Practice

PREVIOUS EXPERIENCE:

- Office Manager – Metropolitan Life Insurance Company, Healthcare Division
- Medical Office Manager – Albany Medical Center, Urological Group
- Dental Office Insurance Clerk – Dr. Leon Jackson (general practitioner)

RELATED SKILLS:

- Recently completed six-month certificate course in dental assisting
- Good "people" skills; great team player
- Excellent bookkeeping and computer skills
- Reliable, honest, hard worker
- Flexible; able to handle multiple tasks simultaneously
- Organized and business-minded
- Positive attitude and great smile
- Raised and educated three children

Figure 15-2.   Sample functional résumé.

inquiry (seeking employment), the job desired (office manager), and the source of the notification (*Albany Times Union*). The cover letter should also state availability for employment (starting date available, e.g., upon graduation, May 30th), and how to be reached to schedule an interview or for further information (current/future telephone number) (Figure 15-3).

May 28, 2_____

Dr. Avery Miller
Buffalo Orthodontic Associates
123 Wolfe Rd., Suite 607
Buffalo, NY 14226

Dear Dr. Miller:

I read with great interest your recent advertisement in *The Buffalo Evening News* for an office manager.

I am a recent graduate of Niagara Community College Dental Assisting Program and would like the opportunity to interview with you for this position.

In addition to formal training, I worked as a chairside dental assistant after school and during summer vacation for Dr. Frank Engle, of Batavia.

During my externship at Niagara County Community College, I had the opportunity to work in several different dental offices, including the orthodontic practice of Dr. Henry VanEsse. I thoroughly enjoyed working in this specialty and I love working with children.

I will be available following graduation and sitting for the National DANB credentialing testing (after June 5th of this year) , and can be reached at: (716)555-3344. Enclosed is a copy of my résumé. If further information is required, please don't hesitate to contact me.

Thank you for your consideration.

Sincerely,

Sarah Jessica Dean
Enc: Résumé

Figure 15-3.   Sample cover letter.

Preparing for the Interview

The **interview** takes place when the two or more parties meet face-to-face to discuss the nature of the job and to obtain additional information from each other. Occasionally, the interview may involve several or all of the dental team members. Group interviews provide an ideal environment to assess the ability of the candidate to function as a team member.

In some practices, part of the interview may include personality profile testing to determine traits and characteristics of the applicant.

In preparing for the interview it is important to make a good first impression. This includes wardrobe, professional demeanor, interviewing skills, and follow-up.

Appropriate Dress and Professional Demeanor

The wise candidate plans to dress conservatively, according to local conventional business dress codes. For women, this generally means a conservative suit (no shorter than mid-kneecap), white or light pastel blouse, neutral hose, and low, closed toe and heel pumps. *Note: the office manager should not wear a uniform or scrubs to the job interview!* If the office manager is a male, he should wear a dress shirt and tie with conservative business slacks and dress shoes (never athletic shoes!).

A conservative purse or brief case is acceptable. Jewelry and other accessories should be kept to a minimum. A watch and wedding band are acceptable; conservative earrings include a single pearl or small gold posts. Jewelry that makes a noise with any body movement is unacceptable.

Nails should be short and clean, and may be polished with clear or a very light (neutral) color. The free edge of the nail should be no more than 2 to 3mm. Artificial nails or excessively long nails are unprofessional.

The hair style should be professional and away from the eyes, face, and collar. Flamboyant hair accessories should be avoided and the applicant should not have to touch her hair during the interview.

Perfume, cologne, or aftershave should be minimal and the applicant should not smoke, chew gum, or ingest food or drink during the interview. Children should be left at home with appropriate supervision.

Plan Ahead

The organized office manager candidate plans to arrive early for the interview. If unsure of the exact location of the office or parking accommodations, it is acceptable to call the office to request this information, and/or to take a trial drive ahead of time. Many applicants will also welcome the opportunity to freshen up at the office prior to meeting the interviewer/dentist.

Although sometimes unavoidable, car problems and traffic may pose punctuality problems. It is advisable to make sure that reliable transportation is available and that sufficient travel time is planned.

In addition to having forwarded a copy of the résumé, the office manager should bring an extra copy or two, in the event the interviewer has misplaced the original. Having an extra copy allows the candidate the opportunity to review the information included, as a refresher and to answer specific questions regarding the information contained in the résumé. Because the candidate may be asked to complete an employment application prior to being interviewed, she or he should also be prepared and bring along a pen.

During the Interview

Because first impressions are all-important, the office manager candidate should remember to walk, speak, and sit professionally. It is appropriate to introduce oneself and to extend the right hand to give a firm handshake upon arrival. Always smile, nod, and exude a positive attitude!

Maintaining good eye contact and composure ensures a confident professional appearance. The candidate should pay attention to the interviewer's questions and give only appropriate responses to them. Refrain from giving additional information or from asking probing questions until the end of the interview or until the interviewer asks, "Do you have any further questions?"

The office manager candidate should also avoid nervous mannerisms, such as finger drumming, nail biting, or repetitive movement of the feet or legs. Speak in a low, but direct voice, avoiding shrill noises and excessive laughter.

The candidate should not bring up the matter of financial compensation and benefits; the interviewer should address this, as well as the open starting date and other pieces of information crucial to the nature of employment. However, the candidate should bring this up should the interviewer overlook it.

The interview may be conducted by one person or several representatives of the practice. The candidate may be invited back to undergo a "working interview," in which specific tasks are walked through with the candidate actually participating in office management tasks, or at a minimum being asked, "How would you handle this?"

Information That May Not Be Discussed

Specific personal information may not be requested by an employer, such as marital status, number of children, racial origin, creed, spouse's employment, personal financial indebtedness, or lifestyle preference (see *Chapter 2, Legal and Ethical Issues and Responsibilities* for additional information regarding EEOC guidelines).

Authorization to Release References and Other Information

In some states it is illegal to release employment information without a person's consent. The interviewer may request information such as references from previous employers, college transcripts, and other information pertinent to past employment history.

To avoid confidentiality issues, the prospective interviewer may ask the employment candidate to sign a waiver, granting release of this information or requesting permission to contact these parties. *Note that personal information or information not relevant to the specific nature of employment may not be requested!*

Generally, information that may be legally given includes start and end dates of employment, the name of the direct supervisor, the job title, and the nature of the job duties.

Drug Testing

The issue of drug testing as a preemployment requirement is becoming more common. It is considered legal in most states and is designed to protect the practice, as well as the patients.

After the Interview

The employment candidate should let the interviewer conduct or lead the interview, and also close it. The candidate should not appear rushed, nor should she or he consume too much of the interviewer's valuable time.

Upon completion of the interview, the candidate should stand, extend her or his right hand for a closing handshake and thank the interviewer, using her or his name.

Upon returning home, the office manager candidate should prepare a follow-up thank-you letter to the interviewer/dentist. The follow-up letter should be brief and recap impressions of the interview (Figure 15-4).

June 6, 2____

Howard Garvalone, DDS, PC
2990 Elmwood Ave.
Troy, NY 19973

Dear Dr. Garvalone:

What a pleasure it was to meet you last Tuesday to discuss the office manager position. I was especially impressed with the office, including your pleasant staff, the attractive decor and the open operatory environment. Everyone at your office made me feel so comfortable, I can see why you have a thriving practice. Just being there made me feel as though I would like to become a patient!

If you have further questions or would like additional information, please do not hesitate to contact me. I can be reached most afternoons and evenings at: (518) 555-3377.

Thank you for the opportunity.

Sincerely,

Dorothy L. Ward, CDA

Figure 15-4. Sample follow-up thank-you letter.

Terms of Employment

Once employment has been secured, it is important for the office manager and employer to establish clear communication regarding all aspects of the position. This includes, but is not limited to, the nature of the job, including a detailed job description, the hours, compensation, benefits, and other office policies.

Letter of Employment

Some practices issue a letter of employment, which serves as a written document outlining the terms of employment. A letter of employment clarifies the terms of the position for both employer and employee and serves as documentation of the employer's expectations.

Information may include duties and responsibilities, working/office hours, salary and benefits, uniform requirements and dress code, provisional employment, and continuing education guidelines.

Provisional Employment

Some employers establish provisional employment following a successful interview. Provisional employment, formerly referred to as a probationary period, provides a time for the prospective employee and the employer to work together, with the end result that a satisfactory employment agreement is met for permanent employment. Provisional employment is further described in *Chapter 2, Legal and Ethical Issues and Responsibilities.*

Salary Negotiations

Generally, the salary is predetermined by the dentist-employer. However, in some instances, there may be specific needs or requests of the office manager that may be negotiated once the job offering has been made.

Other Career Opportunities in Dentistry

In addition to traditional employment in a dental office, there are many other employment opportunities for the dental assistant. In recent years, the trend in these jobs has grown.

Teaching

The experienced dental assistant/office manager may have the desire to share her or his knowledge and skills with others and may thus desire to pursue a teaching career. Most post-secondary dental teaching institutions require a minimum of DANB Certification, a specific number of years of experience working in a dental office, and a baccalaureate degree; or, the teaching candidate must be working toward a four-year degree.

Sales: Retail Supply Houses, Dental Manufacturers, and Telemarketing Organizations

Some former dental assistant/office managers who especially enjoy a fast-paced working environment, travel, and being with the public may secure employment in dental sales. Sales positions require attention to detail and working on a salary-plus-commission basis.

Outside sales opportunities arise from retail dental supply houses and from dental manufacturers who distribute through retail supply houses. Often, dental sales representatives exhibit a company's products at dental trade shows and may also visit schools to give product demonstrations.

Inside sales positions may entail telemarketing promotions to dental offices.

Dental Consultant

Many dental office managers with previous experience may wish to join consulting offices or open their own dental consulting businesses. If considering opening a business, it is advisable to obtain additional information about the legal and financial considerations of self-employment.

Dental School Clinics

There are more than 50 dental schools in the United States, with openings for clinical dental assistants, clinical supervisors, supply and dispensing assistants, and instrument processing assistants. These jobs are especially advantageous to working parents with children at home during school vacations.

Government Clinics, Public Health, and Correctional Facilities

Government-funded clinics serve a variety of the population's needs. They may be funded by county, state, or federal agencies and generally provide basic dental services or prepare statistical reports on dental health status and treatment needs for underserved populations.

Public health departments, usually funded by the state, may provide a source of alternative employment for the experienced office manager. Correctional facilities are owned privately or by the state or federal government. Working conditions are rigid and the environment includes private camera surveillance and security officers.

State Board of Dental Examiners

Occasionally, state dental boards have clerical, licensing, enforcement, investigative, and special service officer positions open. Former dental assistants/office managers may find these positions especially interesting, due to their dental background and familiarity with dental procedures. These positions are available through state employment.

Insurance/Managed Care Corporate Offices

The rapid increase in third-party organizations and managed care have created a need for data input people, claims reviewers, and supervisors. Because of their familiarity with dental terminology and procedures, dental assistants/office managers may find these positions of interest.

Skill-Building for Success: Student Activities

These optional activities and exercises are designed to help the student put into practice information learned in the chapter.

1. Prepare a résumé (either chronological or functional) that best describes your marketable skills. (Estimated working time 60 minutes)

2. Using a fictitious dentist's name and address, prepare a cover letter, stating your desire for employment and availability. (Estimated working time 20–30 minutes)

3. Taking turns with classmates, role play a job interview as an office manager. Be prepared with questions about the job description, starting date, and nature of the position.

4. Using the same fictitious dentist's name and address, prepare an interview follow-up thank-you letter.

Skills Mastery Assessment: Post-Test

Directions: Select the response that *best* answers each of the following questions. Only one response is correct.

1. The trend toward solo, fee-for-service practices is increasing.

   a. True
   b. False

2. The office manager may find employment in:

   a. private, general, solo, fee-for-services practices
   b. group practices and managed care facilities
   c. specialty practices
   d. any/all of the above

3. Many classified advertisements are run as blind ads to ensure confidentiality of the employer/dentist.

   a. True
   b. False

4. Electronic job searches:

   a. increase speed of inquiry
   b. save on postage and paper
   c. allow employers to scan résumés into a database for instant retrieval
   d. all of the above

5. Campus placement offices do all of the following *except:*

   a. charge a fee for applicant screening
   b. post ongoing job openings for students and alumni
   c. match students with employers in the area
   d. operate at no cost

6. Employment agencies are privately owned or franchised companies that:

   a. prescreen and pretest applicants
   b. work on a flat-fee or commission basis
   c. save screening time and administrative costs for the dentist/employer
   d. all of the above

7. A résumé contains all of the following *except*:
   a. a review of the candidate's credentials and qualifications for employment
   b. the candidate's biographical information
   c. a follow-up thank-you letter to the interviewer
   d. the education and previous work experience pertinent to desired employment

8. The two types of résumés are:
   a. revisional and organizational
   b. organizational and chronological
   c. revisional and functional
   d. chronological and functional

9. A résumé should always be printed out on bright colored paper to catch the interviewer's attention.
   a. True
   b. False

10. A résumé should be geared toward a specific job.
    a. True
    b. False

11. The office manager should always include present/previous salary information on a résumé.
    a. True
    b. False

12. A cover letter:
    a. introduces the candidate
    b. explains the reason for the inquiry
    c. states the specific job desired and availability for employment
    d. all of the above

13. To make a professional impression, the office manager should wear a clinic jacket or scrubs to the interview.
    a. True
    b. False

14. To become an instructor, most post-secondary dental teaching institutions require all of the following *except:*

   a. DANB Certification
   b. a specific number of years of experience working in a dental office
   c. registration as a dental hygienist
   d. a baccalaureate degree or evidence of working toward a four-year degree

15. The rapid increase in third-party organizations and managed care have created a need for data input people, claims reviewers, and supervisors.

   a. True
   b. False

16. Employment in a dental school may be especially advantageous to working parents because most require evening employment.

   a. True
   b. False

17. A résumé should always include:

   a. references
   b. Social Security number
   c. spouse's occupation
   d. none of the above

18. A résumé should always include specific contributions or improvements made in a previous position.

   a. True
   b. False

19. A sales position in the dental field may include in employment in any of the following *except:*

   a. a retail dental supply house
   b. a dental manufacturing company
   c. a dental association
   d. a telemarketing organization

20. One should include the present employer's telephone number on a résumé.

a. True

b. False

References

Dietz, E. Polishing up your résumé. *Dental Assisting Magazine.*

Evans, S. (1997, Fall). Getting to and through the interview. *Preview.*

Half, R. (1990). How to write a better résumé. In How to get a better job in this crazy world. : Crown Publishers.

Kern, D. (1993, January). Properly handling reference requests. *Dental Economics.*

Answer Key

Chapter 1

1. D	11. D
2. B	12. D
3. D	13. A
4. B	14. D
5. A	15. B
6. D	16. A
7. D	17. D
8. A	18. D
9. D	19. D
10. C	20. A

Chapter 2

1. D	11. C
2. A	12. D
3. D	13. A
4. B	14. D
5. D	15. D
6. D	16. D
7. E	17. C
8. B	18. B
9. C	19. A
10. C	20. E

Chapter 3

1.	D	11.	D
2.	D	12.	D
3.	A	13.	C
4.	A	14.	D
5.	D	15.	D
6.	D	16.	D
7.	B	17.	D
8.	C	18.	D
9.	D	19.	A
10.	A	20.	D

Chapter 4

1.	D	9.	B
2.	C	10.	D
3.	B	11.	C
4.	C	12.	B
5.	A	13.	D
6.	D	14.	B
7.	A	15.	C
8.	B	16.	D

Chapter 5

1.	B	9.	A
2.	D	10.	A
3.	B	11.	D
4.	D	12.	D
5.	A	13.	C
6.	A	14.	A
7.	D	15.	A
8.	D	16.	B

Chapter 6

1. D		7. A	
2. D		8. C	
3. D		9. D	
4. C		10. B	
5. B		11. D	
6. A		12. D	

Chapter 7

1. B		11. B	
2. C		12. D	
3. D		13. D	
4. B		14. A	
5. D		15. B	
6. C		16. C	
7. B		17. D	
8. C		18. D	
9. D		19. A	
10. C		20. A	

Chapter 8

1. D		11. D	
2. B		12. A	
3. A		13. B	
4. C		14. B	
5. D		15. A	
6. B		16. D	
7. C		17. D	
8. D		18. C	
9. D		19. A	
10. A		20. B	

Chapter 9

1.	A	11.	A
2.	D	12.	D
3.	C	13.	B
4.	D	14.	C
5.	B	15.	D
6.	B	16.	A
7.	D	17.	B
8.	B	18.	C
9.	A	19.	B
10.	C	20.	D

Chapter 10

1.	D	11.	B
2.	B	12.	C
3.	D	13.	B
4.	C	14.	A
5.	A	15.	B
6.	A	16.	D
7.	C	17.	D
8.	D	18.	A
9.	A	19.	B
10.	D	20.	C

Chapter 11

1.	D	10.	C
2.	B	11.	A
3.	D	12.	B
4.	C	13.	D
5.	B	14.	B
6.	D	15.	A
7.	A	16.	D
8.	D	17.	A
9.	A	18.	D

Chapter 12

1. D		11. B	
2. A		12. A	
3. B		13. B	
4. C		14. B	
5. B		15. D	
6. A		16. A	
7. D		17. D	
8. C		18. C	
9. D		19. A	
10. B		20. D	

Chapter 13

1. A		11. B	
2. D		12. C	
3. A		13. D	
4. C		14. D	
5. D		15. A	
6. C		16. A	
7. C		17. D	
8. A		18. D	
9. D		19. D	
10. D		20. C	

Chapter 14

1. C		11. A	
2. B		12. D	
3. B		13. D	
4. A		14. A	
5. B		15. C	
6. D		16. A	
7. A		17. A	
8. D		18. D	
9. D		19. B	
10. B		20. D	

Chapter 15

1.	B	11.	B
2.	D	12.	D
3.	B	13.	B
4.	D	14.	C
5.	A	15.	A
6.	D	16.	B
7.	C	17.	D
8.	D	18.	A
9.	B	19.	C
10.	A	20.	B

Glossary

A

abandonment – failure to provide necessary dental treatment.

accounts payable – the system of distributing money owed by the practice.

active abuse (domestic) – any act of violence within the home that may result in physical trauma, especially about the head and neck.

advertising – the promotion of products or services provided by a business or organization through a variety of media.

amenities – gestures of comfort or convenience.

anatomic dental chart – shows the anatomic landmarks of the teeth and some supporting oral structures.

anomaly – any deviation from the normal.

anterior – toward the front.

anterior sextant – comprises the six front teeth in each arch (jaw).

anxiety – a normal but enhanced feeling of concern.

appointment card – a courtesy to remind patients of their next appointment. It typically contains the business card information on one side and the specifics of the appointment on the reverse.

automatic payment system – a system whereby the payor's bank automatically deducts a specific amount owed to a third party.

B

backorder – occurs when an item ordered is not in stock with the vendor/supplier and will be shipped separately to the dentist's office when it becomes available.

bicuspid/premolar – a permanent tooth having two cusps. The adult dentition contains a first and second bicuspid/premolar in each quadrant.

bid – an offer extended to a number of suppliers to provide all dental supplies at a lower price.

biofilms – microorganisms that accumulate on surfaces inside moist environments such as dental unit waterlines, allowing bacteria, fungi, and viruses to multiply. This can significantly increase a patient's susceptibility to transmissible diseases.

biohazard warning label – a label or tag affixed to hazardous waste items; it must be readable from a distance of five feet.

block/unit appointment scheduling – specific units of time allocated for scheduling dental appointments; most often 10- or 15-minute units.

Bloodborne Pathogens Final Standard – an OSHA regulation that covers all dental employees who could *reasonably anticipate* coming into contact with blood, saliva, and other potentially infectious materials (PIMs) during the course of employment.

buccal/facial – the surface facing *toward the cheeks* in the posterior region of the mouth; it is named for the buccinator (chewing) muscle.

business card – a marketing device that contains all of the information found on the letterhead stationery in a condensed size.

byte – computer memory that corresponds to one location, usually capable of storing one character.

C

call list – a handy reference for the office manager to fill an opening in the appointment schedule on short notice.

capitation – a form of contracted care, usually by a corporation, institution, or other group; the provider receives a set fee per patient per a given timeframe and provides all or most of the services covered in the program to subscribers.

case presentation – a non-treatment appointment when the dentist or office manager meets with the patient (and often an accompanying family member) to explain an extensive case.

Cash on Delivery (COD) – a form of cash payment for minimal expenditures of the practice.

Centers for Disease Control and Prevention (CDC) – a federal agency that sets guidelines for healthcare practitioners; CDC's guidelines are enforced by OSHA.

Certified Dental Assistant (CDA) – a dental assistant who has completed the requirements for certification through the Dental Assisting National Board.

child abuse – an act of physical violence or negligence of care of a minor within the home.

code of ethics/ethics a moral obligation that encompasses professional conduct and judgment imposed by the members of a particular profession; considered a higher standard (moral) than jurisprudence (legal) requirements.

compensation – financial remuneration in the form of wage, salary, or paid benefits.

consumable supplies – those that are completely used up or consumed with use.

contract – an agreement with one vendor to purchase all the office's supplies in return for the lowest bid on the total supply budget for the year.

coordination of benefits – submitting dual coverage claims according to the instructions provided by two insurance companies.

copayment – the portion of a healthcare charge that must be paid by the patient, stated as a flat amount.

cover letter – accompanies a résumé; introduces the candidate and explains the reason for the inquiry, the job desired, and the source of the notification.

credit invoice – a credit or refund issued against a statement.

crown – a prosthetic replacement of the coronal portion of a natural tooth; a crown may be three-quarter or full.

D

deciduous/primary dentition – the first set of teeth, consisting of 10 teeth in each arch. The deciduous dentition is eventually replaced by the secondary (succedaneous) or permanent dentition.

Dental Assisting National Board (DANB) – the national credentialing organization for dental assistants.

dental hygienist – a member of the dental team whose primary duties include the prevention of dental disease. The dental hygienist must be licensed in the state of employment.

dental laboratory technician – a member of the dental team who fabricates crowns, bridges, dentures, and orthodontic appliances.

dental radiograph (X-ray) – An image of the tooth, teeth, mouth, jaws, and/or related oral structures on film.

dental supply representative – a salesperson who provides the office with new products, information, and services to help the practice run smoothly.

dentin – the layer of tooth surface below the enamel; it comprises the bulk of the tooth and determines tooth shade.

denturist – a dental professional who takes impressions of the oral cavity and fashions full and partial dentures for patients; some states require licensure to work as a denturist.

diagnosis – the clinical conclusion reached by the dentist resulting from an oral examination and review of additional aids including radiographs, study models, periodontal disease susceptibility, and the intraoral camera.

digital radiography or radiovisiography – a computerized method of projecting and freezing dental radiographic images onto a computer screen for examination and storage in a database.

direct marketing campaign – a specific promotion directed to a defined target audience.

direct reimbursement – a self-funded program in which the individual patient or employee is reimbursed based upon a percentage of dollars spent for care provided; it allows beneficiaries to seek treatment from the provider of their choice.

direct supervision – duties legally delegated by the dentist to be performed by qualified staff; the dentist must be physically present in the office while these duties are performed.

disk/diskette – a secondary storage device that stores information or data to be input for processing or "installed" for a specific function; a disk is also used as a back-up device.

distal – the surface facing away (distant) from the midline of the mouth, following the line of the arch.

double-book – a method of appointment scheduling in which two patients are booked at approximately the same time; it is commonly used for patients who are chronically late or likely to disappoint.

dual coverage – a system of insurance participation that permits spouses who both carry dental insurance to cover each other as dependents, increasing the amount of the benefit up to the actual cost of the treatment.

E

edentulous – having no natural teeth.

elder abuse – an act of physical violence or negligence of care of a person 65 years or older within the home or care facility.

electronic charting – the chairside assistant directly inputs all clinical findings of the dentist into the treatment room computer.

electronic funds transfer – transfer of funds from one account to another, usually via the telephone.

embezzlement – the fraudulent appropriation of money entrusted into one's care.

emergency patients – patients of record or first-time patients who call the office in pain or for an unforeseen urgent visit, who do not have an appointment.

enamel – the hardest structure in the human body; forms the outer covering of the crown of the tooth.

endodontics – the field of diagnosis, cause, prevention, and treatment of diseases of the dental pulp and related tissues.

endodontist – a dental specialist who performs root canals and related procedures.

engineering controls – specific equipment or devices that facilitate prevention of accidental exposure.

Environmental Protection Agency (EPA) – regulates and registers certain products used in dental practices, including surface disinfectants; requires products to undergo and pass specific testing requirements prior to approval for registration.

equipment – major items that are used for five or more years and may be depreciated by the office over a number of years.

esthetics – a pleasant or cosmetic appearance.

event marketing – a form of internal marketing that acknowledges specific events or occasions according to information contained in the individual patient's attribute profile.

expendable supplies – those items that are relatively low in cost and are replaced frequently.

exposure-control plan – identifies tasks, procedures, and job classifications where occupational exposure takes place.

exposure incident – specific eye, mouth, or other mucous membranes, nonintact skin or parenteral (through the skin) contact with blood or other PIMs that directly results from the performance of an employee's duties.

external marketing – marketing efforts or campaigns directed to people outside of the office who may desire to become patients.

extraction – surgical removal of a tooth; an extraction may be classified as either simple or complicated.

F

facial/labial/facial – surface that faces toward the face or lips.

Fédération Dentaire Internationale System – the tooth numbering system that combines quadrant number as the first digit with the tooth number in the quadrant as the second digit; this tooth numbering system designates tooth #11 through #48 in the adult dentition and tooth #51 through #85 in the primary dentition.

filing systems – either manual or computerized; a system of office records management.

fixed bridge – a prosthetic replacement for one or more missing teeth.

fixed expenses – office overhead expenses which remain approximately the same from month to month.

flagging system – a device used to alert the office manager that it is time to reorder a supply product.

focus group – a small group or representative cross-section of the patient base.

Food and Drug Administration (FDA) – a federal agency that regulates marketing of medical devices, including equipment and disposable items; it also reviews product labels for false or misleading information and sufficient directions for use.

G

general supervision – duties legally allowed to be performed by qualified staff; the dentist need not be physically present in the office while these duties are performed, but should be available by telephone or pager.

geometric dental chart – depicts the teeth as round graphic elements with lines differentiating the surfaces and edges.

H

handicap – any neurologic or physical disabilities that impair function. Neurological handicaps may be motor, sensory, emotional, or intellectual in nature. Advanced age and obesity do *not* qualify as impairments under the *AwDA.*

hardware – physical or visible computing equipment.

hazard communication program – a written program outlining the methods and procedures used in the office to reduce risks to staff associated with hazardous substances, diseases, chemicals, or PIMS.

Hazard Communication Standard – the *Employee Right to Know Law,* which addresses the right of every employee to know the possible dangers associated with hazardous chemicals and related hazards in the place of employment; this law also requires employers to provide methods for corrective action.

Hepatitis B vaccination – must be provided by the employer to all full-time employees who may have potential for occupational exposure; the dentist must provide this at no charge to employees.

I

impacted (tooth) – a tooth locked in the jawbone.

impairment – any physiological disorder or condition, cosmetic disfigurement, or anatomical loss; or any mental or psychological disorder, such as mental retardation, emotional or mental illness, or specific learning disabilities.

incisal edge – the biting edge of the anterior teeth.

incisor – anterior tooth used for biting and cutting.

information packet – provides a number of pieces of information about the practice.

injury/accident log – must be kept on file to reflect occupational exposure incidents and corrective/follow-up methods.

input device(s) – consisting of the keyboard and/or mouse, the input devices interpret commands in a manner that allows the computer to process specific information.

inscription – the portion of a pharmaceutical prescription that contains the name of the drug, dosage form, and the amount of the dose.

insured party – any person covered under the insurance plan.

internal marketing – promotional efforts targeted to existing (active) patients of the practice.

interview – when two or more parties meet face-to-face to discuss the nature of the job and to obtain additional information from each other.

intraoral camera – a computerized device that uses a wand inside the mouth to enlarge dental images onto a color monitor, print color photographs, or film a video of an oral examination.

inventory – a written or computer-printed list of all supplies on hand, the amount ordered, the manufacturer/supplier, and the per unit price.

invoice – a statement requesting payment for merchandise purchased.

J–K

job description – a written list of duties to be performed by an employee.

jurisprudence – a set or system of laws; dental jurisprudence is set forth by each state's Legislature in the Dental Practice Act.

L

label – the part of the prescription that describes the contents.

letterhead stationery – paper and envelopes imprinted with the logo, name of the practice (if used), the doctor's name and credentials, the office address, telephone number, and fax number; if the office is on-line, it may also contain the practice's *e-mail address* or *website address*.

liable/liability – being held legally responsible for an act.

licensee – the holder of license to perform specific duties within the dental office, issued by the State Board of Dental Examiners. The dentist and dental hygienist must be licensed in the state in which they perform dental procedures.

lingual – the tooth surface facing toward the tongue.

logo – a design or symbol that represents a business.

M

malpractice – professional negligence; failure to perform one's professional duties, either by omission or commission.

managed care – a cost-containment system that directs the utilization of health benefits by restricting the type, level, and frequency of treatment; limiting access to care and controlling the level of reimbursement for services.

mandible – the lower jaw.

marketing – creating the need or demand for, or awareness of, a product or service the consumer may have been unaware was available, or that he or she may have been unaware that he or she desired; dental practices may ethically promote their services through a variety of internal and external marketing strategies.

Material Safety Data Sheets (MSDSs) – written information about the content and potential hazard of specific products used in the dental office. Each product that has a potential hazard must have a corresponding MSDS on file in the office.

maxilla – the upper jaw.

media – forms of advertising including telephone directories, newspapers, magazines, radio, television broadcasting, and billboards.

medical waste – liquid or semi-liquid body fluid, including any items in the dental office that release *bioburden* when compressed; items caked with dried body fluid that have the potential to release bioburden during handling; contaminated sharps; and pathological and microbial wastes containing body fluid.

mesial – tooth surface facing *toward the midline* of the mouth.

molar – a posterior tooth; the adult dentition has three molars in each quadrant.

N

National Practitioner Data Bank – established in 1986 as a national reporting entity to track and monitor complaints against licensed healthcare professionals, including dentists and dental hygienists.

negligence – performing something that a reasonable professional would not do, or not doing something a reasonable professional would.

newsletter – communicates information about the practice and the services it provides; it may also profile interesting developments and advances in dental techniques and treatments and offer professional advice to patients.

non-compliance – failure to adhere to laws, rules, or regulations set forth in the State Dental Practice Act.

O

occlusal – the chewing surface of the posterior teeth.

occupational exposure – an exposure incident which involves accidental contact with blood or other PIMS that directly results from the performance of an employee's duties.

Occupational Safety and Health Administration (OSHA) – a government agency that enforces guidelines for protection of workers; OSHA has federal, regional, and state offices.

on-line – hooked up with a server on the internet; having access to individuals and organizations via *e-mail addresses* or *website addresses.*

operating system – system software program that co-ordinates the hardware capabilities of the computer.

operatory – the treatment room where dental procedures are performed.

oral pathologist – a dental specialist who studies diseases and conducts research related to the oral cavity.

oral pathology – the field of diagnosis and treatment of oral disease that may affect the entire body.

oral prophylaxis – cleaning, scaling, and polishing of the teeth; a preventive dental procedure.

oral surgeon – a dental specialist who extracts teeth, removes diseased tissue, surgically exposes impacted teeth, wires fractured jaws, and places dental implants; a maxillofacial surgeon may also treat victims of automobile accidents or disease (for example, cancer), who require reconstruction of facial features and tissues; also orthognathic surgery.

oral surgery – the field of diagnosis and treatment of diseases and malformations of the oral cavity and surrounding structures.

Organization for Safety and Asepsis Procedures (OSAP) – a national organization of teachers, practitioners, dental healthcare workers and manufacturers/distributors of dental equipment and products; it focuses on developing and communicating standards and information on aseptic technology to dental practices and educational institutions.

output device(s) – the equipment that translates the information from the CPU into a format that can be read by the user; may be a *monitor* (screen), a *printer,* or *speaker(s).*

overhead – the operating expenses associated with running the dental practice.

overtime pay – awarded to hourly wage earners who work beyond the standard 40 hours per week.

P

packing slip – a piece of paper identical to the original order and subsequent invoice for payment due; the packing slip is shipped with the merchandise.

pager – a cordless electronic device to which a caller directs a specific telephone number for a call to be returned; the pager activates with a buzzing or vibrating sound or motion.

paid leave – compensated time away from the office, including holidays, vacation, and sick time.

palliative – treatment offered to relieve immediate pain only.

Palmer system – the tooth numbering system that designates teeth by quadrant; the adult (permanent) dentition starts with #1 as the central incisor through the third molar, which is #8; the primary (deciduous) dentition starts with letter A as the central incisor through the second deciduous molar, which is letter E. Specific quadrants are indicated by brackets.

passive abuse (domestic) – a form of neglect to care for a family member.

patient attributes – specific information about a patient; date of birth, hobbies, names of family members, etc.

patient base – the total number of active patients in the practice.

patient education brochures – describe oral conditions and the need for preventive, restorative, postoperative, or corrective treatment.

patient profile – a list of characteristics, attributes, or information about a patient.

pediatric dentist (formerly *pedodontist*) – a dental specialist who treats children from their first dental visit through approximately age 18.

pediatric dentistry (formerly *pedodontics*) – the field of treatment of children's teeth.

performance review – a review by the dentist-employer (or in large practices the office manager) of an employee's employment performance; usually conducted annually.

periodontal – the area around the tooth.

periodontal ligament – acts as a shock absorber to cushion the tooth in the socket and provides attachment to the jawbone.

periodontics – the field of preserving natural tooth structures through disease prevention and treatment of the support tissues around the teeth.

periodontist – a dental specialist who performs gingival (gum) treatments, including surgery, exposure of oral implants, and occlusal (chewing) adjustments.

periodontium – tissue surrounding the tooth.

permanent/secondary/succedaneous dentition – the second or adult set of teeth; a full complement comprises 32 teeth.

petty cash voucher – a tangible receipt as proof of cash monies paid for office expenses.

phobia – subject to or suffering from irrational fear.

porcelain-fused-to-metal – a single crown or multi-unit bridge that is made with porcelain on the outside and metal on the inside.

posterior – toward the back.

Potentially Infectious Materials (PIMs) – substances and contaminated objects that have potential to cause cross-contamination in the dental office; blood and saliva and items contaminated with them are the most common PIMs.

practice goals – an extension of the practice philosophy and mission statement; may be broken down into written, measurable outcomes.

practice mission statement – a succinct declaration of the practice philosophy, usually formulated into one or two sentences.

practice philosophy – the theme that drives the practice on a daily basis.

practice survey – a survey designed to solicit feedback from patients for improvement of services and office amenities.

primary dentition – see deciduous dentition.

probe systems – devices used to automatically calculate periodontal pocket depths and record this information into a computer data base.

production scheduling – a philosophy and system of scheduling for maximum productivity.

prognoses – anticipated or expected treatment outcomes; *prognosis* is the singular form.

prostheses – artificial teeth or appliances that replace or repair existing natural teeth.

prosthodontics – the field of restoration and maintenance of normal dentition and its functions through replacement with artificial teeth; one of the eight dental specialties.

prosthodontist – a dentist who has received additional postgraduate training following completion of dental school to replace lost natural teeth with fixed or removable prostheses.

protocol – from the same root as in "prototype," protocol refers to an accepted form or format, usually for behavior in a specified professional or social situation; protocol in a dental practice refers to the accepted and standard way of doing things.

provider – the person or entity providing direct patient care and to whom third-payment is released; the dentist.

provisional employment – temporary employment, usually for 90 days, that implies permanent employment upon completion of a satisfactory trial period.

public health dentistry – the field of study, prevention, and treatment of dental diseases through community, county, state, and federal programs and agencies.

proximate cause – a directly contributing action that results in an undesirable outcome.

public health dentist – a dental specialist who provides dental services to a variety of population groups under the sponsorship of a community- or government-sponsored agency or program.

pulp – provides the blood and nutritional supply from the body to the tooth; the pulp enters each tooth through the apical foramen.

purchase order – a specific document used for supply purchases and repair requisitions.

purchase order number – a specific number assigned to each purchase or repair requisition.

Q

quadrant – one quarter of the mouth; the deciduous quadrant comprises five teeth; the primary quadrant comprises eight teeth.

R

rate of use – the rate of consumption of items and supplies commonly used in the office.

recall card – a printed reminder of a return visit for preventive dental care, usually issued every six months.

recall program – once a patient has completed current necessary treatment he or she will be "recalled" to the practice at some time in the future for an oral examination, prophylaxis, and any subsequently required radiographs or treatment; the most common recall interval is six months.

references – names of people who could provide a job recommendation; these are usually former employers.

referral – a recommendation made by one person to another; a recommendation for professional treatment.

refill – the part of the prescription where the dentist indicates the number of refills (if any) allowed.

reorder point – a predetermined minimum quantity of a specific supply left in inventory; when the item reaches the minimum quantity additional units are to be ordered to avoid running out.

responsible party – the person who accepts the financial responsibility for paying the dental fee. If this person is not the patient, it is usually a parent, guardian, or a spouse. For insurance purposes, the patient must be a covered claimant on the responsible person's policy, but if there will not be any insurance participation in the fee, there are no restrictions. Anyone can sign an agreement to pay for the patient's care. These exceptions are typically a companion other than a spouse, or an older sibling who is not actually the legal guardian of a minor patient.

restrictive endorsement – special conditions or restrictions limiting the receiver of the check concerning use that can be made of the check.

résumé – a review of the employment candidate's credentials that states his or her qualifications for employment; it contains the candidate's biographical information, type of employment sought, and education and previous work experience pertinent to desired employment.

risk management – strategies taken by the dentist and staff to prevent or reduce the likelihood of a patient bringing legal action.

S

shelf life – the amount of time a product is guaranteed fresh; a product should be used before the shelf life expires or it should be discarded.

signature on file – the insured's signature kept on file by the office manager to facilitate processing of claims.

solo practice – an office run and owned by one dentist.

spousal abuse – any form of physical violence or neglect by a partner or significant other within the home; sometimes referred to as *battered woman syndrome.*

standard of care – treatment guidelines that a dentist with the same knowledge, skill, and care in the same community would provide; there are no absolutes in standard of care.

State Board of Dental Examiners – the regulatory body that maintains and enforces the rules and regulations of the State Dental Practice Act and issues dental licenses; it is charged with protecting the health, safety, and welfare of the public.

State Dental Practice Act – a written set of rules and regulations governing the legal conduct of dental licensees within each state.

statement – the primary means by which a practice receives compensation from patients for services provided.

study models – stone or plaster casts of the patient's teeth and supporting structures.

subscription – the portion of the prescription that contains the amount of the drug and directions for preparation of the drug for dispensing.

succedaneous dentition – the secondary dentition, which succeeds the primary dentition.

superscription – the portion of a pharmaceutical prescription that contains the date of the prescription, the patient's name, address, age, and gender.

supplier/vendor – a company through whom the dental office orders supply items used in the office.

system unit – the electronic circuitry housed within the computer cabinet; it performs the memory and processing functions of computer processing.

T

target audience – a segmented, predetermined group of people, based upon specific criteria or attributes.

target mailing – a promotional mailing piece directed toward a specific group of people called a target audience.

temporomandibular joint (TMJ) – the only joint in the head; it connects the mandible to the cranium.

termination – discontinuation of employment or dismissal of a patient.

treatment code – a specific number assigned to each scheduled procedure.

treatment plan – A complete diagnosis, including recommended treatment and sequence of scheduled visits.

U

unerupted (tooth) – a tooth that has formed but has not appeared in the oral cavity.

universal precautions – treating all patients as having a potentially infectious disease.

universal system – a tooth numbering system adopted by the American Dental Association in which the teeth of the permanent dentition comprise #1 through #32; the teeth of the primary dentition comprise letters A through T.

unprofessional conduct – any act or deed that fails to uphold the State Dental Practice Act.

V

variable expenses – overhead expenses associated with the practice that change from month to month.

voice-activated dental charting – a computerized system of dental charting whereby the operator verbally dictates the clinical findings of the exam into the practice's data base.

voice mail – a recorded message service that intercepts the line after a set number of rings and asks the caller to leave a message; with a simple voice-mail system, the call will not be answered if the line is busy.

voice messaging – a telephone answering system that automatically answers the call with a recorded message; it provides further instructions for the caller to leave a message or stay on the line for operator assistance.

W–Z

walk-out statement – a statement of the individual patient's services and charges, amount paid (if any), and remaining balance (if any).

work practice controls – changing the way procedures are currently performed to ensure a higher degree of safety or protection from accidental exposure.

Index